NUTRITION AND WEIGHT CONTROL FOR LONGEVITY

Lora Brown Wilder, Sc.D., M.S., R.D.,

Lawrence J. Cheskin, M.D.,

and

Simeon Margolis, M.D., Ph.D.

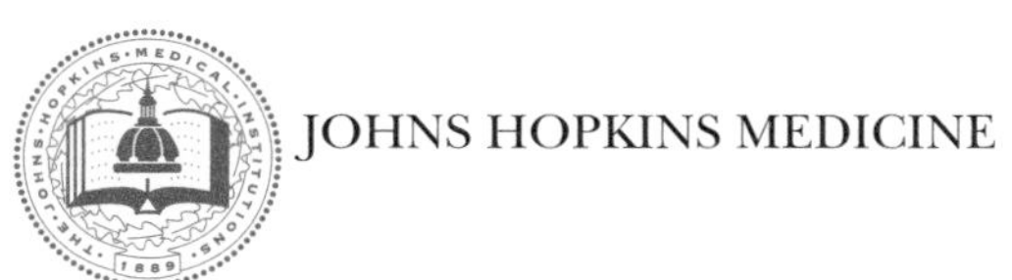

Dear Reader:

Eating right not only contributes to your everyday health and energy, but also is key to longevity. A diet that provides you with nutrient-rich foods can be a powerful tool in preventing life-shortening conditions—including obesity, which has reached epidemic proportions in the United States. Maintaining a healthy diet—and using diet in combination with exercise to maintain a healthy weight—can help lower the risk of high blood pressure, heart disease, diabetes, osteoporosis, and many kinds of cancer. This White Paper provides the very latest findings on nutrition and disease prevention, and offers expert, practical guidance on how to enjoy a health-promoting diet and lose unwanted pounds.

Here are some of this year's highlights:

- What **everyday activities** can help you lose weight? (page 72)
- You know calcium is good for your bones, but how about **vitamin D**? (page 24)
- Are **artificial sweeteners** safe to eat? (page 66)
- Do you have a **food allergy** or a **food intolerance**? The difference is important. (page 38)
- Weighing the risks and the benefits of **soy**. (page 10)
- New research: a **dietary key** to reducing your risk of ischemic stroke. (page 31)
- The diet that **lowers cholesterol** as effectively as drugs. (page 8)
- Being overweight may increase your risk of developing **Alzheimer's disease**. (page 68)

We are hopeful that the guidelines and advice in this White Paper will serve as a blueprint for a lifetime of healthful eating and weight control.

Sincerely,

Lora Brown Wilder, Sc.D., M.S., R.D.
Assistant Professor
Johns Hopkins School of Medicine

Lawrence J. Cheskin, M.D.
Director
Johns Hopkins Weight Management Center

P. S. Don't forget to visit www.HopkinsAfter50.com for the latest health information that will complement your Johns Hopkins White Paper.

THE AUTHORS

Lora Brown Wilder, Sc.D., M.S., R.D., a registered dietitian, received her M.S. in nutrition from the University of Maryland and her Sc.D. in public health from Johns Hopkins University. She is currently an assistant professor at the Johns Hopkins University School of Medicine and is also affiliated with the United States Department of Agriculture and the University of Maryland's Department of Nutrition and Food Science. Dr. Wilder has served on various advisory committees related to nutrition, including committees at the American Heart Association and the National Institutes of Health, and helped set up the first Johns Hopkins Preventive Cardiology Program. In her research, Dr. Wilder has studied the effects of coffee on fatty acids and investigated behavioral strategies to reduce coronary risk factors. Her current research is in the area of dietary assessment methodology. She contributed to *Nutritional Management: The Johns Hopkins Handbook* and has been published in *Circulation, The American Journal of Medicine,* and *Journal of the American Medical Association.*

■ ■ ■

Lawrence J. Cheskin, M.D., graduated from Dartmouth Medical School and completed a fellowship in gastroenterology at Yale-New Haven Hospital. Currently, he is an associate professor of international health and human nutrition at the Johns Hopkins Bloomberg School of Public Health and an associate professor of medicine at the Johns Hopkins University School of Medicine. Dr. Cheskin is also the director of the Johns Hopkins Weight Management Center. In his research, Dr. Cheskin has studied the effects of medications on body weight, the gastrointestinal effects of olestra, how cigarette smoking relates to dieting and body weight, and the effectiveness of lifestyle changes in weight loss and weight maintenance. He is also the author of four books: *Losing Weight for Good, New Hope for People with Weight Problems, Better Homes and Gardens' 3 Steps to Weight Loss,* and *Healing Heartburn.* Dr. Cheskin has appeared on television news programs and lectured both professional and lay audiences on the topics of weight loss and management.

■ ■ ■

Simeon Margolis, M.D., Ph.D., received his M.D. and Ph.D. from the Johns Hopkins University School of Medicine and performed his internship and residency at Johns Hopkins Hospital. He is currently a professor of medicine and biological chemistry at the Johns Hopkins University School of Medicine and medical editor of *The Johns Hopkins Medical Letter: Health After 50.* He has served on various committees for the Department of Health, Education and Welfare, including the National Diabetes Advisory Board and the Arteriosclerosis Specialized Centers of Research Review Committees. In addition, he has been a member of the Endocrinology and Metabolism Panel of the United States Food and Drug Administration.

CONTENTS

NUTRITION AND WEIGHT CONTROL FOR LONGEVITY

Eating right will help you maintain a healthy weight and may protect you against a variety of chronic diseases, including coronary heart disease (CHD), cancer, diabetes, and osteoporosis. Most people recognize the importance of a healthy diet, and yet they do not always follow one. A recent report issued by the Congressional General Accounting Office notes that only 23% of Americans get their recommended servings of fruit and only 41% get their recommended servings of vegetables.

People cite a multitude of obstacles to practicing good nutrition: time constraints, the ready availability of packaged and processed foods, the perception that they will have to give up their favorite foods, and confusion over conflicting information on nutrition and weight loss. And many people harbor the misguided belief that dietary changes made late in life are of little consequence. In fact, changing dietary habits and losing weight in middle or even old age can significantly influence health. This White Paper addresses these concerns and counters them with simple, effective strategies for achieving good nutrition and, in particular, keeping your weight under control.

Nutrition

This section of the White Paper gives an overview of nutrition principles and specific recommendations—based on research studies—for the intake of various nutrients.

THE BASICS OF NUTRITION

Food provides not only the energy we need to function but also the nutrients required to build all tissues (such as bone, muscle, fat, and blood) and to produce substances used for the chemical processes that take place in our bodies millions of times a day. There are two broad categories of nutrients: macronutrients (carbohydrates, protein, and fats), which supply energy and are needed in large amounts to maintain and repair body structures; and micronutrients, the vitamins and minerals required in small amounts to help regulate chemical processes. Fiber, technically not a nutrient, also is part of a healthy diet.

Calories (technically called kilocalories) are the measure of the amount of energy in a food. One calorie represents the amount of heat needed to raise the temperature of 1 L of water by 1° C. Carbohydrates and protein contain four calories per gram; fat contains nine calories per gram; alcohol contains seven calories per gram.

Carbohydrates are starches and sugars obtained from plants. Sugars are known as simple carbohydrates and starches as complex carbohydrates. All carbohydrates are broken down in the intestine and converted in the liver into glucose, a sugar that is carried through the bloodstream to the cells, where it is used for energy. Some glucose is converted into glycogen, which is stored in limited amounts in the liver and muscles for future use. Carbohydrates are converted into fat when intake exceeds immediate needs and glycogen storage capabilities.

Proteins are nitrogen-containing substances that make up muscles, bones, cartilage, skin, antibodies, some hormones, and all enzymes. The proteins in foods are broken down in the intestine into amino acids, the building blocks for body proteins. The body can manufacture 13 of the 22 amino acids present in proteins; these 13 are called nonessential amino acids because they need not be obtained from the diet. The other nine are known as essential amino acids because they must be supplied by food.

Fats belong to a group of substances called lipids and are made up of chains of carbon, hydrogen, and oxygen that vary in length and in the number of hydrogen atoms attached to the carbon atoms. All fats are combinations of saturated and unsaturated fatty acids. The degree to which a fatty acid is loaded with hydrogen determines its "saturation" and impact on health. Along with protein and carbohydrates, fat is one of the three nutrients that supply calories to the body. Fat is vital for the proper functioning of the body. For example, fats are used to store energy in the body, insulate body tissues, and transport fat-soluble vitamins through the blood.

Vitamins are organic substances (meaning that they contain carbon) needed to regulate metabolic functions within cells. Vitamins do not supply energy, but one of their functions is to aid in the conversion of macronutrients into energy. Fat-soluble vitamins (A, D, K, and E) are stored in the body for long periods, whereas water-soluble vitamins (the B vitamins and vitamin C) can only be stored for a short time (although vitamin B_{12} is stored for longer periods). See the chart on pages 20–21 for the functions of the individual vitamins.

Minerals are inorganic substances that serve many functions, including helping to maintain water content and acid–base balance (pH) in the body. Macrominerals (calcium, phosphorus, chloride, sodium, magnesium, potassium, and sulfur) are present in the body in large amounts. Microminerals, though no less important, are present in smaller amounts. The most important minerals and their functions are listed in the chart on pages 28–29.

Fiber is present in fruits, vegetables, grains, and legumes. Suppling no nutrients or calories, fiber is not digestible, but it is valuable in speeding foods through the digestive system and (possibly) binding toxins and diluting their concentration in the intestine. Some types of fiber also help to control blood sugar and blood cholesterol levels.

Water is an essential nutrient because it is involved in all body processes. Since an individual's water needs vary with diet, physical activity, environmental temperature, and other factors, it is difficult to pin down an exact water requirement. The general recommendation is to drink at least six to eight 8-oz. glasses of water daily, which can be accomplished by drinking water as well as other fluids (broth and fruit juice) and by eating foods that contain a large percentage of water (fruits, vegetables, and soups).

Cholesterol is a waxy, fat-like substance that is produced mainly in the liver but can also be made by any cell in the body except red blood cells. The liver produces all the cholesterol the body needs, but cholesterol is also found in any animal product you eat, such as meats, poultry, fish, eggs, butter, cheese, and milk. (Plant foods contain no cholesterol.) For transport in the blood, cholesterol associates with certain proteins to form lipoproteins. Cholesterol is present in the membranes of all cells, acts as insulation around nerve fibers, and serves as a building block for some hormones.

FAT

By now, almost everyone is aware that reducing dietary fat can lessen the risk of several chronic diseases. While a high fat intake contributes to obesity, CHD, and some forms of cancer, not all types of fat have the same effects on health.

Triglycerides are the most abundant fats in foods as well as in the body's fat cells and are the body's main source of stored energy. Triglycerides are manufactured in the liver and fat cells as well as obtained from food. It takes about eight hours for all of the triglycerides ingested during a meal to be removed from the blood where, like cholesterol, they are transported on lipoproteins.

The Rewards of Eating Vegetarian

A plant-based diet has compelling health benefits. At the same time, it can require planning to get the optimal balance of nutrients.

The American Dietetic Association (ADA) asserts that vegetarian diets are healthful, nutritionally adequate, and provide benefits for the prevention and treatment of certain diseases. Studies show that vegetarians have reduced risks of heart disease, high blood pressure, type 2 diabetes, obesity, and some types of cancer.

How do vegetarian diets produce these health benefits? Generally lower in total fat, saturated fat, and cholesterol, they help decrease blood cholesterol levels. In addition, plant foods contain compounds that interfere with the actions of carcinogens (cancer-causing chemicals), help repair damaged cells, and alter levels of hormones involved in cancer development. They also provide ample fiber, which may lower the risk of heart disease, stroke, diabetes, and gastrointestinal cancers.

Do Vegetarians Get Enough Protein?

Proteins are composed of amino acids—substances that the body needs for growth and for the maintenance of muscles, tendons, ligaments, and other tissues. Although many amino acids are manufactured in the body, nine "essential" amino acids can only be obtained from food. A food protein that supplies all of the essential amino acids is called a complete protein (animal foods are sources of complete protein). A food protein that does not supply all the essential amino acids is called an incomplete protein.

Plant proteins (with the exception of soy protein) are incomplete. But if the sources of dietary protein are varied, plant foods alone can supply enough of the essential amino acids—especially if the diet regularly includes high-protein plant foods such as beans, lentils, nuts, nut butters, and whole-grain breads and cereals. In addition, certain combinations—for example, rice and beans, or corn and beans—form complete proteins. And while it's not necessary to eat these food combinations at the same meal, they should be consumed over the course of a day.

Soy foods contain especially high-quality protein. In fact, soy protein (found in soybeans, edamame, tofu, tempeh, soy nuts, and soy milk) contains enough of all the essential amino acids to be considered a complete protein equal in quality to proteins of animal origin.

Nutrient Needs for Strict Vegetarians

While a vegetarian diet is healthful, strict vegetarians (vegans) may be deficient in certain nutrients—such as vitamin B_{12}, vitamin D, calcium, iron, and zinc—that are found principally in animal products. Careful food choices and use of a multivitamin supplement can help prevent nutritional deficiencies caused by strict vegetarian diets.

Vitamin B_{12}. Found in such animal foods as fish, dairy, eggs, meat, and poultry, vitamin B_{12} is required to maintain healthy nerve cells, to produce red blood cells, and to make DNA, the genetic material in all cells. As we age, our ability to absorb vitamin B_{12} diminishes. In fact, some experts estimate that 10% to 30% of older adults do not absorb vitamin B_{12} efficiently from food.

Because they eat no animal foods, strict vegetarians are at risk for developing a deficiency of this important vitamin, especially if they also eat few B_{12}-fortified foods (such as fortified cereals). For this reason, it is a good idea for vegetarians—particularly those who are over the age of 50—to take a vitamin B_{12} supplement.

Vitamin D. This vitamin is vital for maintaining proper calcium balance, which is necessary for bone and muscle health and other functions. Mostly produced by the body

Triglycerides can be any combination of three types of fatty acids—saturated, monounsaturated, and polyunsaturated—which differ in their chemical structures. As a result, no food contains just one type of fatty acid. Instead, the fat in a particular food is classified as saturated or unsaturated based on the type of fatty acid that predominates. For example, olive oil is typically thought of as a monounsaturated fat, but it also contains some polyunsaturated and saturated fat: 75% of the oil is monounsaturated, 14% is satu-

through exposure to sunlight, vitamin D is also found in some foods, principally fatty fish and fish oils, as well as certain fortified foods, such as some brands of soy milk, cereal, cow's milk, and orange juice.

Studies show that the diets of many vegetarians, particularly vegans, contain inadequate amounts of vitamin D. And though lacto-ovo-vegetarians probably get enough vitamin D, and vegans can get vitamin D from fortified foods, it is still a good idea for them to consult their physician or a registered dietitian about supplementation. (For more information, see "Are You Getting Enough Vitamin D?" on page 24.)

Calcium. This mineral is essential for numerous functions, including regulation of the heartbeat, conduction of nerve impulses, stimulation of hormone secretions and blood clotting, as well as for building and maintaining healthy bones. Because lacto-ovo-vegetarians consume dairy foods, their calcium intakes are comparable to or higher than those of nonvegetarians. However, the calcium intakes of vegans are generally lower than those of either lacto-ovo-vegetarians or omnivores.

Good plant sources of calcium include bok choy, broccoli, napa cabbage, collards, kale, okra, and turnip greens. In addition, vegans may find it easier to meet their calcium needs by including fortified foods in their diets. Foods fortified with calcium include certain brands of orange juice and apple juice, breads, cereals, soy milk, and tofu. If you are concerned about your calcium intake, consult your physician about taking calcium supplements.

Iron. Adequate iron intake is necessary to prevent anemia. Because the richest dietary sources of iron are red meat and liver, vegetarians have a greater risk of iron deficiency than nonvegetarians. Although plant foods can contain iron, it's a type of iron ("nonheme" iron) that is not absorbed as well as the "heme" iron contained in meat. In addition, the absorption of nonheme iron can be inhibited by certain substances in plant foods such as fiber, phytates (in cereal grains), and oxalates (in green leafy vegetables).

Nonheme iron can be absorbed better if a source of vitamin C is eaten at the same time as the iron-containing food. Good nonmeat sources of iron include dried beans, peas, whole-grain breads, spinach, enriched products, nutritional yeast, and dried fruits. Plants foods that are a good source of vitamin C include citrus fruits and juices, strawberries, tomatoes, broccoli, bell peppers, cooking greens, and potatoes.

Zinc. This essential mineral supports a healthy immune system and is required for DNA synthesis. It is also needed for wound healing, as well as maintaining your sense of taste and smell. Zinc is most abundant in animal foods, and although the mineral is present in certain plant foods—such as whole grains, wheat germ, fortified cereal, nuts, and legumes—its bioavailability appears to be lower in vegetarian diets.

Vegetarians may need as much as 50% more zinc than nonvegetarians because of the lower absorption of zinc from plant foods; so it's very important for vegetarians to consume high-quality sources of zinc on a regular basis. In addition, most multivitamins contain enough zinc to help make up for any deficiencies in a vegetarian diet.

Vegetarian Lexicon

While all vegetarian diets place plant-based foods on center stage, the extent to which animal products are avoided can vary. For example:

- Vegans (pronounced VEE-gans), also called strict, pure, or total vegetarians, eat only plant foods; they avoid all products derived from animals (including honey).
- Ovo-vegetarians allows eggs in addition to plant foods.
- Lacto-ovo-vegetarians allow dairy and eggs in addition to plant foods.
- Pesco-vegetarians don't eat red meat, but do eat fish, eggs, and dairy.
- Semi-vegetarians don't eat red meat, but do include poultry, fish, eggs, and dairy.

rated, and 9% is polyunsaturated. (The percentages do not add up to 100% because other fat-like substances also are present in the oils.)

Fatty acids serve crucial functions in the body: They are required for the membranes of cells, keep skin and hair healthy, and form triglycerides that provide a layer of insulation under the skin. Since the body cannot manufacture them, certain fatty acids must be obtained from foods and are therefore called essential fatty acids. They are required components of cell membranes and can be converted to important hormone-like substances. In addition, dietary fat is needed to help the intestine absorb the fat-soluble vitamins A, D, and E.

Saturated fatty acids carry all the hydrogen atoms that their carbon chains can hold. Saturated fats are solid at room temperature and are found in abundance in animal products, such as meats, cheese, milk, and butter. Tropical oils—palm, palm kernel, and coconut—are also saturated. Saturated fats raise blood cholesterol levels and possibly contribute to certain forms of cancer.

Monounsaturated fatty acids are missing one pair of hydrogen atoms. As a result, two neighboring carbon atoms form what is known chemically as a double bond. The "mono" in monounsaturated indicates that these fatty acids have just one double bond. Liquid at room temperature, they predominate in foods such as olive oil, canola oil, almonds, and avocados. Cholesterol levels drop when monounsaturated fats replace saturated fats in the diet.

Researchers discovered the value of monounsaturated oil in part by studying the Mediterranean diet, which is associated with low rates of CHD and, possibly, cancer, despite a relatively high total fat intake. Olive oil is the main source of fat in that diet. The Mediterranean diet is also high in fruit, vegetables, and grains. This relatively low intake of animal foods may also account for the diet's heart-healthy effects. (See page 35 for new research that further confirms the healthful nature of the Mediterranean diet.)

Polyunsaturated fatty acids have two or more ("poly," meaning many) double bonds. Also liquid at room temperature, polyunsaturated fats make up the majority of the fatty acids in safflower, sunflower, and corn oils; in fish; and in some nuts, such as walnuts. Most of the polyunsaturated fats in plants are called omega-6 fatty acids, because the last of the double bonds is located at the sixth carbon atom in the fatty acid chain.

Fish contains both omega-6 fatty acids and another type of fatty acid called omega-3. Researchers believe that two specific omega-3 fatty acids, eicosapentaenoic acid (EPA) and docosahexaenoic acid (DHA)—found primarily in seafood—may help reduce blood pressure and prevent cardiac arrhythmias (abnormal heart rhythms). Small amounts of omega-3 fatty acids are also found in vegetable sources such as walnuts; and soy, canola, and flaxseed oils. While they appear to have some of the benefits of omega-3 fatty acids in fish, more research is required to determine their benefits.

All polyunsaturated fats lower blood cholesterol levels when substituted for saturated fats in the diet.

Dietary Fat and Coronary Heart Disease

A diet high in saturated fats increases CHD risk by raising blood cholesterol levels. Body cells use fat as an energy source and need cholesterol as a component of their membranes. Because fat is not soluble in the watery environment of the bloodstream, the liver wraps the cholesterol and triglycerides in a layer of proteins to transport them through the blood. These protein-wrapped packages are called lipoproteins, of which there are three main types:

Very low density lipoprotein (VLDL) carries triglycerides from the liver to other cells. As the triglycerides are removed from VLDL, they are converted into smaller, cholesterol-rich particles, called low density lipoproteins (LDL). Often referred to as "bad" cholesterol, LDL is first oxidized before it is taken up by cells in the arterial walls, where it initiates a series of changes that result in the formation of atherosclerotic plaques. These plaques can eventually hinder blood flow in arteries throughout the body. The formation of a blood clot on the plaques can halt blood flow altogether: Blockage of an artery supplying the heart causes a heart attack, while a blockage in an artery leading to the brain leads to a stroke.

The third type of lipoprotein is called high density lipoprotein (HDL). As it travels through the bloodstream, HDL helps reduce the buildup of arterial plaque by removing cholesterol from arterial walls and returning it to the liver for disposal. For this reason, HDL cholesterol is often called "good" cholesterol.

Measures to prevent the formation of plaques include reducing blood levels of triglycerides and LDL cholesterol while raising HDL cholesterol. The different types of fatty acids in foods have varying effects on the levels of LDL and HDL cholesterol. Saturated fatty acids increase levels of LDL cholesterol, while diets low in saturated fats reduce LDL levels. Although not everyone responds to the same degree, on average, every 1% reduction in saturated fat calories reduces total blood cholesterol levels by about 2 mg/dL, mostly from a decrease in LDL cholesterol. Saturated fats raise LDL levels by reducing LDL's removal from the blood by the liver. Polyunsaturated fats overcome this effect by reducing the amount of saturated fat in the diet.

Blood cholesterol levels are also raised by dietary cholesterol, but not as much as by saturated fat. A few foods—egg yolks, lobster, and shrimp—are especially high in dietary cholesterol.

Another type of fatty acid, trans fatty acid (TFA), is formed when food manufacturers add hydrogen atoms to unsaturated fats to make them more saturated and therefore more solid and shelf-

NEW RESEARCH

Size of Cholesterol Particles Possible Key to Longevity

A number of studies have suggested that living an unusually long time—well into one's 90s or past 100—has a strong genetic component. But identifying specific markers and genes that promote longevity in humans has been difficult. Recently, however, researchers pinpointed a biological mechanism that may help prevent or delay the diseases responsible for most deaths.

Researchers studied 213 exceptionally long-lived, healthy, genetically homogeneous Ashkenazi Jews (average age 98 years) and 216 of their children (average age 68 years); they were compared with two age-matched control groups. A crucial finding in the long-lived subjects and their offspring was significantly larger LDL and HDL particles than in the controls. The size of the particles was independent of the absolute blood levels of LDL and HDL cholesterol. Large LDL particles are thought to cause less damage to blood vessels than small particles, which may account for the lower prevalence of cardiovascular disease, hypertension, metabolic syndrome, and diabetes observed in the long-lived subjects.

Further study in this area, conclude the authors, "may provide key insights into preventive and therapeutic interventions" for these major diseases.

JOURNAL OF THE AMERICAN MEDICAL ASSOCIATION
Volume 290, page 2030
October 15, 2003

stable. The American Heart Association recommends cutting down on trans fats, which are used in many packaged cookies, crackers, and other baked goods; commercially prepared fried foods; and most margarines. A report recently issued by the Institute of Medicine (IOM) concludes that there are no safe levels of trans fats. The IOM recommends reducing TFA consumption to as little as possible to decrease risk of heart disease, cancer, and gastrointestinal disorders. Studies suggest that trans fats are even more harmful to health than saturated fats because trans fats not only raise LDL cholesterol, but also lower HDL cholesterol levels more than saturated fats. Elevated levels of blood triglycerides, which are especially common in people with diabetes, may also increase CHD risk.

Eating fish is associated with a reduced risk of CHD. This benefit may be due to special effects of the omega-3 fatty acids found in fish or may simply reflect the fact that many people who eat fish tend to eat less red meat. A growing body of research shows that omega-3 fatty acids may protect against sudden cardiac arrest and irregular heart rhythms. Omega-3s are believed to make blood platelets less sticky and thus less likely to form blood clots that can cause heart attacks. Furthermore, omega-3 fatty acids can also help lower triglyceride levels and decrease blood pressure slightly in people with hypertension. It should be noted, however, that fish oils in capsule form do not lower blood cholesterol levels, although these supplements can reduce triglycerides in people with very high triglyceride levels.

In addition, consuming foods that contain naturally occurring plant compounds called plant sterols (also known as phytosterols) can help lower cholesterol levels and may reduce the risk of CHD. Plant sterols, the ingredients responsible for the benefit of these products, are chemically similar to cholesterol. When they are ingested, the body mistakes them for cholesterol and tries to absorb them without success. As a result, the absorption of cholesterol is partially blocked.

Plant sterols are present in all plant foods but are particularly concentrated in vegetable oils, including corn and sunflower oil. Chemically modified phytosterols are added to certain margarines (as well as other products, such as orange juice, which are currently being formulated to include plant sterols). When used properly, these products, such as the butter substitutes Benecol and Take Control, can help lower LDL cholesterol. The amount of saturated, unsaturated, and trans fat found in each of these products is comparable to regular tub margarine (and none contains cholesterol).

NEW RESEARCH

New Diet Similar to Drugs for Cholesterol Lowering

A vegetarian diet high in sterols, soy, fiber, and almonds can achieve low density lipoprotein (LDL) cholesterol lowering comparable to that achieved with a low-dose statin and better than a low-fat diet, a new study shows.

The study randomized 46 people with high LDL cholesterol to one of three four-week treatments: 1) a vegetarian control diet emphasizing whole grains and low-fat dairy products; 2) the control diet plus 20 mg of lovastatin (Mevacor) daily; or 3) an investigational vegetarian diet emphasizing sterols (natural plant compounds), soy protein, soluble fiber (mainly from oats, barley, psyllium, eggplant, and okra), and almonds.

LDL cholesterol decreased significantly more in the investigational-diet group and the lovastatin group (29% and 31%, respectively) than in the control group (8%). (Higher doses of or more potent statins can lower LDL cholesterol by 50%.) Levels of C-reactive protein, a marker for inflammation and a heart-disease risk factor, decreased significantly less in the control group (10%) than in the investigational-diet group and medication group (28% and 33%, respectively).

Cholesterol guidelines recommend consuming 25 g of soluble fiber daily and possible inclusion of 2 g of plant sterols daily. Levels of intake of soy and nuts have not been established, but these foods have potential heart benefits.

JOURNAL OF THE AMERICAN MEDICAL ASSOCIATION
Volume 290, pages 502 and 531
July 23/30, 2003

One and a half tablespoons of Benecol daily or one to two tablespoons of Take Control can lower total cholesterol by up to 10%. The effect is cumulative when the spreads are used with other cholesterol-lowering measures. Sterol products should be used in place of—rather than in addition to—butter or traditional margarine. Consuming more than the recommended amount will not lower cholesterol more than 10%. A week's supply costs about $5.

Dietary Fat and Weight

Fat is a concentrated source of calories—it has nine calories per gram, compared with four calories per gram in protein and carbohydrates. Small amounts of fatty foods, therefore, pack a lot of calories. Reducing fat intake, however, does not guarantee weight loss. Weight is ultimately determined by the total number of calories consumed—whether from fat, carbohydrates, or protein—and the total number expended by metabolism, daily activity, and exercise. Overeating even fat-free foods can result in weight gain if they are also high in calories.

A low-fat diet that is also low-calorie and is combined with regular exercise will help people maintain an appropriate weight, or lose weight if necessary. Weight loss is the most effective way to lower elevated triglyceride levels. It also helps to raise HDL cholesterol levels: In one study, a 5-lb. weight gain lowered HDL levels by 4% in men and by 2% in women; losing weight counteracts this effect. Weight loss is also the first line of treatment for type 2 diabetes. In addition, a weight loss of as little as 5 to 10 lbs. may lower blood pressure enough to make antihypertensive drugs unnecessary. The many factors that affect weight control—and healthy strategies for losing weight—are discussed in detail in the section beginning on page 48.

Dietary Fat and Cancer

As with CHD, the hypothesis that a high-fat diet promotes the development of certain cancers first came from observational studies of different populations. In cultures where fat consumption is low, such as Japan and China, rates of breast, colon, ovarian, and prostate cancer are also low. In countries where people eat high-fat diets—the United States and Finland, for example—the incidence of these cancers is high. Furthermore, as people emigrate from a country where a low-fat diet is the norm to one where a high-fat diet predominates, and they adopt the dietary habits of their new homeland, their rates of these cancers increase. Thus, some researchers

The Benefits and Risks of Soy

Should you be eating more soy? The answer is yes, but with some caveats.

Soy foods and supplements are derived from soybeans, a legume that has been a staple of Asian diets for centuries. Low in saturated fat and cholesterol free, a mere ½ cup of cooked soybeans provides a wealth of nutrients—thiamin, riboflavin, vitamin B_6, folate, fiber, iron, potassium, magnesium, selenium, and vitamin E. Soybeans are also chock-full of phytochemicals (plant chemicals), most notably isoflavones, which are a type of phytoestrogen (a plant hormone akin to human estrogen).

Along with this impressive roster of nutrients and phytochemicals, soybeans (and products derived from them) have a unique protein content. Unlike other legumes, soybeans are a source of "complete protein," meaning they contain all of the amino acids necessary for building and maintaining tissue in the body.

Furthermore, the protein in soy is naturally bound to its isoflavones: One gram of soy protein is attached to approximately 2 mg of soy isoflavones. This is significant because studies suggest that naturally bound soy protein and isoflavones confer more health benefits than either substance alone. Isoflavones added to soy foods (that is, not naturally bound to soy protein) or in supplement form (that is, without any soy protein) may not have the same health benefits. For more information about the isoflavone content of different soy foods, see the inset box.

Soy and Heart Health

Eating foods containing soy is consistent with American Heart Association dietary guidelines that call for limiting animal fat and consuming more nuts, fruits, and vegetables. When substituted for animal protein in the diet, soy protein lowers total and LDL cholesterol and triglycerides without lowering HDL cholesterol. In a recent randomized, controlled study, adults with high cholesterol experienced significant improvements in LDL cholesterol (as well as C-reactive protein, a substance in the blood associated with heart disease) after one month of eating a diet rich in cholesterol-lowering foods, such as soy (see the sidebar on page 8).

The U.S. Food and Drug Administration permits food manufacturers to state that consuming 25 g of soy protein a day lowers the risk of coronary heart disease. Manufacturers can print this health claim on the labels of soy-based foods if the product contains at least 6.25 g of soy protein per serving and is low in cholesterol and fat. The claim cannot be printed on soy protein supplements, because specific disease claims are not permitted for supplements.

Just how soy lowers cholesterol is unclear. Some studies suggest that soy helps sweep LDL cholesterol out of the bloodstream and into the liver, an effect that may be triggered by soy's two major isoflavones. However, researchers are still unsure which components of soy are responsible for its cardiovascular benefits. Compelling evidence does indicate that a combination of both soy protein and soy isoflavones is necessary to achieve the greatest cholesterol-lowering effects from soy.

Soy may provide additional cardiovascular benefits. Preliminary evidence suggests that it may help to reduce blood pressure, possibly by improving the elasticity of blood vessels. In one recent, double-blind, randomized study, 40 adults with mild to moderate high blood pressure experienced moderate improvements in blood pressure after drinking 4 cups of soy milk each day for three months. Promising research suggests that the substances in soy may also exert beneficial antioxidant actions on blood vessels.

Soy and Cancer

According to population-based studies, breast and prostate cancer rates

believe that the fat content of the diet, rather than differences in the genetic makeup of people from different countries, is responsible for the increased cancer risk.

Animal studies supported the link between dietary fat and cancer, but human studies have produced conflicting results. While some studies have shown that total fat intake is directly related to cancer risk, others have suggested that a high calorie intake, a diet rich in red meat, or a high intake of saturated fats may be the causative factor. Still other research shows that even if total fat in-

Isoflavones in Soy Foods
The amount of isoflavones in soy foods depends on how it was processed. For example, while 1 cup of soy milk provides about 24 mg isoflavones, 1 cup of cooked soybeans will give you almost four times that amount (95 mg).

To preserve isoflavone content when cooking soy at home, experts recommend keeping cooking time to a minimum by adding soy foods, such as tofu and miso, late in the cooking process. At right is a list of soy foods with their respective amounts of isoflavones in milligrams per serving.

Food	Isoflavones (mg)
Soybeans, dried, cooked (1 cup)	95
Soybean sprouts (¼ cup)	57
Soy nuts (¼ cup)	55
Natto (½ cup)	52
Tempeh (4 oz.)	50
Soy flour, full-fat (⅓ cup)	49
Tofu, firm (4 oz.)	28
Soy milk (1 cup)	24
Edamame,* cooked (4 oz.)	16
Miso (2 tablespoons)	15

*edible green soybeans

are lower in countries where soy consumption is high. While some laboratory and animal studies support soy's protection against these cancers, there has not yet been any definitive evidence from human studies. Soy isoflavones are thought to protect against hormone-dependent cancers of the breast, uterus, and prostate by blocking the actions of certain hormones that stimulate tumor growth. In addition, experimental research has shown that genistein (a major soy isoflavone) may help to detoxify some cancer-causing substances.

Soy's Additional Health Benefits
Preliminary evidence suggests that by exerting estrogen-like effects on the body, soy's isoflavones may relieve hot flashes associated with menopause. And promising findings indicate that both soy protein and isoflavones may inhibit bone loss and thus help prevent osteoporosis. Further, many soy foods are fortified with calcium and vitamin D, two nutrients vital for bone health.

What Are the Risks?
Based on what is presently known, eating a moderate amount of soy foods is beneficial and safe for nearly everyone. For reasons that are still unclear, however, preliminary research shows that phytoestrogens may have both proestrogen and antiestrogen properties, and high doses of isoflavones might cause hormonal imbalances that increase the risk of certain hormone-sensitive cancers.

In summary, a serving or two of soy foods each day is generally fine, but large amounts of soy foods or supplements are inadvisable. Until more is known about soy's relationship to cancer, those with a history of breast cancer are best advised to avoid soy supplements and to discuss the consumption of soy foods with their doctor. Additional research is needed to determine the mechanism of soy's beneficial effects, to be sure they are not outweighed by possible adverse effects from high amounts of soy (particularly in certain individuals).

Consumer Beware
One thing to keep in mind when choosing soy foods is that they are not all created equal. For example, soy foods that are designed to look and taste like meat products (for example, hot dogs or bologna) often have high amounts of sodium. Look for minimally processed soy foods, such as tofu or whole soybeans, because they are low in saturated fat and sodium and have the nutritional attributes currently believed to be responsible for soy's health benefits. To ensure that a food contains substantial amounts of soy protein and isoflavones, check the product label and choose foods that list soy as one of the first three ingredients.

take is not involved in the development of cancer, it can accelerate progression of the disease.

Research into the role of dietary fat in breast cancer is a good example of the conflicting data on fat and cancer risk. Several studies have linked fat intake to breast cancer development, while others have found no connection. One possible explanation is that dietary fat itself does not raise breast cancer risk but does so indirectly by promoting weight gain. Several studies have shown that weight gain in adulthood is associated with an increased risk of developing breast cancer. For example, a Canadian study published in the *International Journal of Cancer* found an association between adult weight gain and breast cancer in older women. Among 1,233 women with breast cancer and 1,237 without the disease, the risk of postmenopausal breast cancer was 35% higher in those who had gained 55 pounds or more before menopause. (For more on weight gain and cancer, see "The Obesity-Cancer Connection" on page 54.)

Alternatively, the fat content of the diet in childhood or early adulthood may determine cancer risk, so changes made in mid- to late life may not appreciably decrease risk.

One difficulty with connecting a high-fat diet to cancer is that no measurable factor in the body can be used to determine the increased risk, as with blood cholesterol levels and CHD, for example. It may be that cancer risk is not reduced until fat intake is very low. Because of the relatively high fat content of typical Western diets, modest reductions in fat intake by participants in U.S. studies may be too small to affect cancer risk.

The method by which food is cooked may play a role in the development of cancer. For example, studies suggest carcinogens, called polycyclic aromatic hydrocarbons, form when the fat from animal foods drips onto hot coals or stones during grilling. The resulting smoke from flare-ups can then transfer these cancer-causing compounds to food.

In addition, studies indicate that the type of fat in the diet may also be significant. In Mediterranean countries, for example, where monounsaturated fats (in the form of olive oil) make up a large part of the diet, women have a lower risk of breast cancer than women in the United States, even though their average total fat intake is about 42% of calories, compared with 35% in the United States. Fats derived from some fish and plant sources (such as avocados, nuts, and seeds), on the other hand, may reduce the risk of cancer. In countries like Japan where the consumption of fatty fish (tuna, mackerel, and salmon) is high, cancer rates (particularly for breast and prostate cancer) tend to be low. It has been suggested that the omega-3 fatty acids found in fish (and in flaxseeds) may stunt tumor growth by "crowding out" harmful fats that seem to spur cancer growth in the cells.

Recommendations for Fat Intake

1. Above all, keep saturated and trans fat intake to 10% of calories or less. People with CHD, diabetes, or elevated LDL cholesterol levels should get less than 7% of their calories from saturated and trans fat. Meats, poultry skin, and whole-milk dairy products contain the most saturated fat. Limit intake of red meat (beef, pork, and lamb) to two or three servings per week, choose lean cuts (see page 66 for more information on lean cuts), and eat small portions (about 3 oz.). Each week have several meatless meals, such as vegetarian chili or pasta with marinara sauce. Choose low-fat dairy products such as fat-free milk, low-fat yogurt, and reduced-fat cheeses. Limit your trans fat intake. Although trans fats are not listed on food labels yet, the tip-off in the ingredient list is the word "hydrogenated."

2. With few exceptions, limit total fat intake to less than 35% of calories. Most people should not reduce fat intake to less than 20% of calories. For those whose fat intakes have exceeded the recommended amount, fat calories should be replaced with ones from complex carbohydrates, with an emphasis on whole grains, vegetables, fruits, and legumes (beans and peas). As much as possible, avoid calories from products that contain a lot of refined carbohydrates, such as sugar and white flour.

The American Heart Association (AHA) recommends a diet that includes less-saturated fats and oils. In general, consuming leafy greens and replacing red meat with fish are good ways to improve fat and oil intake. To reduce your use of cooking oils, take advantage of cooking methods that naturally reduce fat: Bake, broil, grill, roast, poach, microwave, or steam foods instead of frying or sautéing them. If you do sauté, use nonstick pans or a vegetable oil spray. Use vegetable oils and butter only in moderation, and choose monounsaturated oils (such as olive oil and canola) over polyunsaturated. Small amounts of water, wine, or broth can be added instead to prevent foods from sticking. Also, cut down on margarine and salad dressing and, if you use mayonnaise, look for one based on canola oil.

3. Get half your total fat intake from monounsaturated fats. Monounsaturated fats are particularly plentiful in olive oil, canola oil, almonds, walnuts, and avocados. Because these sources are also concentrated sources of total fat, they must be eaten in moderation to maintain a diet containing no more than 35% of calories from fat.

4. Get less than 300 mg of dietary cholesterol per day, and less than 200 mg if you have elevated LDL levels. Although saturated fat raises blood cholesterol levels more than cholesterol from foods, experts still recommend limiting dietary cholesterol.

5. Eat fatty fish at least twice a week. The omega-3 fatty acids in fatty fish appear to have some protective effect, and fish are a good source of protein and are low in saturated fat. Salmon, sardines,

NEW RESEARCH

Fish, Omega-3s May Reduce the Risk of Alzheimer's

Omega-3 fatty acids, which are abundant in fish, reduce the risk of coronary heart disease. Now, a study demonstrates that people who consume omega-3 fatty acids have a reduced risk of developing Alzheimer's disease.

Among 815 older Chicago residents without dementia, those who consumed fish once a week were 60% less likely to develop Alzheimer's disease after four years than people who rarely or never ate fish. For those who ate fish twice weekly, the risk was reduced by 70%.

Fish is a rich source of two types of omega-3s: docosahexaenoic acid (DHA) and eicosapentaenoic acid (EPA). Another omega-3, alpha linolenic acid (ALA), is found mainly in plant oils and nuts, particularly canola, soybean, and flaxseed oils, as well as walnuts.

In the study, the participants completed dietary questionnaires, and the investigators calculated how much of the three omega-3s each person consumed. Most of the protective effect of omega-3s was from DHA. EPA had no significant effect, and ALA reduced the Alzheimer's risk only in people with a genetic predisposition for Alzheimer's.

These results support the recommendation for regular inclusion of omega-3–rich foods in the diet. As in all epidemiological studies, the benefit demonstrated here needs confirmation.

ARCHIVES OF NEUROLOGY
Volume 60, page 940
July 2003

and albacore tuna are all good choices. Omega-3 fatty acids are also found in soybeans, walnuts, flaxseed, canola seeds, and products made from these foods (such as tofu and various oils).

6. Minimize cancer risk while grilling. The American Institute for Cancer Research advises simple measures, such as selecting lean cuts of meat, trimming fat, marinating, precooking, and minimizing fire flare-ups and smoke.

7. Remember that these recommendations need not be followed for each meal or even on a daily basis. It is more important to even out fat intake over the course of a week. If you eat a high-fat lunch, for example, you can compensate by eating a low-fat dinner or a little less fat than usual over the next several meals.

FIBER

For many years, fiber (the indigestible component of plant foods) was thought to be useful only for adding bulk to the diet to prevent constipation. But the shift in the diets of Western societies from ones based on whole grains, vegetables, fruits, and legumes to diets based on meats, refined grains, and processed foods has been associated with an increase in the incidence of CHD and type 2 diabetes; several studies point to a lack of dietary fiber as a primary cause. Some debate has ensued over whether fiber itself has a protective effect or is simply a marker for a healthy diet. But in recent studies, fiber has emerged as an independent factor for the prevention of disease.

Both types of fiber—soluble (sometimes called viscous) fiber, which dissolves in water and forms a gel-like substance, and insoluble fiber, which does not dissolve in water—are important for disease prevention. Most plant foods contain some of each type, but often one or the other predominates. Soluble fiber is found in legumes, barley, oats, and most fruits, while wheat and other whole grains and some vegetables contain insoluble fiber.

The two types of fiber exert different effects in the intestine. Soluble fiber binds bile acids and removes them in the stools. By absorbing many times its weight in water, insoluble fiber increases stool bulk and helps wastes pass more easily and rapidly through the digestive tract.

Fiber and Heart Disease

The connection between fiber and heart disease has focused on the effect of soluble fiber on blood cholesterol levels. In the liver, cholesterol is used to make bile acids. Soluble fiber binds with bile acids in the intestines and removes them in the stool. The liver responds by converting more cholesterol into bile acids. The resulting fall in cholesterol in liver cells leads them to take up more LDL from the blood.

Studies suggest that an increase of 5 to 10 g per day in soluble fiber intake—two to four extra servings of fruits and vegetables—reduces cholesterol levels by about 5%. Other studies have shown that fiber intake directly affects the risk of fatal and nonfatal heart attacks. Other research indicates that soluble fiber is more strongly associated with a reduced risk of heart attack and CHD death than insoluble fiber. However, the effect of soluble fiber on blood cholesterol levels does not fully account for the protective effect of dietary fiber. This finding opens the possibility that fiber may work in additional ways—by affecting the body's use of glucose and insulin, for example, or by reducing triglyceride levels.

Fiber and Diabetes

People with type 2 diabetes, which accounts for 95% of all diabetes, are resistant to the actions of insulin, a hormone that controls the manufacture of glucose by the liver. To compensate, the pancreas must secrete more insulin to allow glucose in the blood to enter cells, where it is used for energy. Diabetes develops if the pancreas cannot keep up with the continual demand for large amounts of insulin. Dietary fiber is thought to help prevent diabetes—as well as make it easier for people with diabetes to maintain good control of blood glucose levels—because it slows the absorption of sugars from the intestine and diminishes the rise in blood glucose following the ingestion of carbohydrates.

Fiber and Cancer

After skin cancer, colon cancer is the second most common cancer in the United States, where diets tend to be high in fat and low in fiber. Rates are much lower in countries where inhabitants consume a high-fiber, low-fat diet. The relationship between colon cancer and fiber was questioned by a 1999 study that tracked approximately 88,000 female nurses over a 16-year period. Surprisingly, the women who ate the most fiber—nearly 25 g a day—were just as likely to develop cancer and adenomas of the colon as those who ate the least fiber (about 10 g per day). Because the study had limitations in its design and because its findings contradict those of several previous studies, the results cannot be considered definitive.

Dietary Strategies for Disease Prevention

Simple changes to your diet that can help prevent and/or manage specific diseases are outlined below.

Because many of these recommendations for dietary changes overlap, even one or two can help protect against several disorders. While there are important dietary recommendations for cancer prevention, the benefits of dietary changes for coronary heart disease (CHD), hypertension (high blood pressure), diabetes, and osteoporosis are based on stronger scientific evidence.

CHD and Stroke

- Limit saturated fat and trans fatty acids to less than 10% of calories (or less than 7% if you have high blood cholesterol levels). You can accomplish this by restricting your intake of the major sources of saturated fat (fatty meats, poultry skin, full-fat dairy products, and tropical oils) and by restricting your intake of hydrogenated fat (found in commercially prepared baked and fried foods and margarines), the major source of trans fatty acids.
- Center your diet around fish, skinless poultry, and plant-based, unprocessed, whole foods, such as whole grains, fruits, vegetables, legumes (such as beans), and nuts.
- Eat at least two servings of fish per week, particularly fatty fish such as mackerel, salmon, and albacore tuna. Fatty fish provide a type of fat, called omega-3 fatty acids, that is believed to be heart healthy.
- Include soy foods in your diet—replace foods high in saturated fat and cholesterol with 25 g of soy protein per day. This recommendation is particularly important for those with high levels of total and LDL cholesterol.
- Opt for fat-free and low-fat dairy products. Also choose lean meats in place of higher-fat cuts. The leanest cuts of meat are loin, flank, and round.
- Get at least 15% of total calories from monounsaturated fats such as olive oil. Choose unsaturated fats instead of saturated and trans fats.
- Limit cholesterol to 300 mg per day. If you have high blood cholesterol levels, limit your intake to less than 200 mg per day.
- Get 20 to 30 g of fiber per day (for adults over age 50); include plenty of soluble fiber.
- Consume at least 400 micrograms (mcg) of folate (folic acid) per day from fruits, vegetables, fortified grains, and/or a supplement.
- Limit intake of refined carbohydrates such as white flour and sugar.
- Maintain a desirable weight to prevent metabolic syndrome, a major risk factor for CHD.

Hypertension

- Maintain a desirable weight.
- Limit daily sodium intake to 2,400 mg, the equivalent of about 1¼ teaspoons of table salt (sodium chloride). To achieve a more dramatic reduction in blood pressure, restrict sodium intake to 1,500 mg or less each day, the equivalent of about ⅔ teaspoon of salt.
- Increase intake of fruits and vegetables to get enough potassium. Aim for eight servings per day.
- Consume two to four servings of fat-free or low-fat dairy products each day for adequate calcium and protein.
- Include plenty of whole grains, fish, and poultry.

While debate continues as to whether a high fiber intake can help prevent breast cancer, some research has shown that dietary fiber may lower blood levels of estrogen, thereby possibly reducing breast cancer risk.

Fiber and Weight Control

A diet rich in fiber helps people control their weight. Studies have found that those who consume fiber-rich diets feel less hungry between meals, get fuller more quickly at mealtime, and tend to consume fewer calories throughout the day.

Fiber-rich foods help to promote feelings of fullness and reduce caloric intake in a variety of ways. Foods high in fiber require more time and effort to chew, so they may reduce the amount of food

- Restrict intake of fat, red meat, and sugary foods and drinks.
- Limit consumption of alcohol to no more than one drink per day for women and no more than two per day for men. One alcoholic drink equals one 12-oz. beer, one 5-oz. glass of wine, or one shot (1½ oz.) of 80-proof spirits.

Osteoporosis

- Consume 1,200 to 1,500 mg of calcium each day.
- Take calcium supplements if the dietary calcium in your diet is low.
- Get an adequate amount of vitamin D (400 to 800 IU per day).
- Limit sodium consumption to 2,400 mg per day.
- Follow a dietary pattern that emphasizes fruits, vegetables, and whole grains.
- Restrict caffeine consumption to less than 300 mg per day. Depending on brewing methods, the average cup (8 oz.) of coffee contains between 115 and 175 mg caffeine; the average size (12 oz.) soda contains between 30 and 50 mg caffeine, depending on the brand.

Type 2 Diabetes

- Maintain a desirable weight.
- Limit saturated fat intake to no more than 7% of total calories.
- Get at least 15% of total fat calories from monounsaturated fat.
- Limit dietary cholesterol to less than 200 mg per day, which requires restriction of all dietary sources of cholesterol, including eggs and shellfish.
- Get at least 25 g of fiber per day; include several servings of whole grains and plenty of soluble fiber.
- Aim for eight servings per day of a variety of fruits and vegetables. At least one vegetable should be dark green and at least one fruit or vegetable should be orange or red.
- Restrict intake of refined carbohydrates such as white flour and sugar.
- Choose an overall balanced diet that emphasizes fruits, vegetables, and whole grains.

Prostate Cancer

- Limit intake of fat from animal sources, especially meats and dairy products.
- Limit your intake of red meat. Choose lean cuts and eat small portions (about 3 oz.).
- Eat a diet rich in whole grains and have at least five servings per day of a variety of fruits and vegetables. At least one of the vegetables should be dark green and at least one fruit or vegetable should be orange or red. Include plenty of cruciferous vegetables, such as broccoli, cauliflower, and cabbage.
- Eat several servings of cooked tomato products (such as tomato sauce) per week.

Breast Cancer

- Maintain a desirable weight.
- Limit fat intake, especially saturated fats and trans fatty acids.
- Get at least 25 g of fiber per day. Be sure to include several servings of whole grains.
- Eat at least five servings per day of a variety of fruits and vegetables. At least one vegetable should be dark green and at least one fruit or vegetable should be orange or red.
- Limit alcohol consumption to fewer than seven drinks per week.

Colon Cancer

- Limit your intake of red meat. Choose lean cuts and eat small portions (about 3 oz.).
- Eat several servings of whole grains and at least five servings of fruits and vegetables each day. Include plenty of spinach, broccoli, tomatoes, oranges, berries, and carrots.
- Get 1,200 mg of calcium per day by eating calcium-rich foods, such as two to three servings of low-fat or fat-free dairy products.

consumed at a meal. The extra time required to chew high-fiber foods produces more saliva, which, along with the extra water that fiber absorbs, is believed to distend the stomach and create a feeling of fullness. Furthermore, dietary fiber is thought to block the absorption of some fat and protein in the intestinal tract, thus reducing the calories derived from these nutrients.

Both soluble and insoluble fiber contribute to weight control in specific ways: Soluble fiber (found in oats, barley, legumes, and dried and fresh fruit) forms a gel around food particles, which slows the passage of food through the stomach and delays hunger signals sent to the brain. Insoluble fiber (found in broccoli, potatoes with their skins, apples, beans, whole-grain breads and cereals) supplies bulk by absorbing water in the digestive tract, which, in turn, contributes to a feeling of fullness and thereby helps to discourage overeating. Consuming the recommended servings of fruits, vegetables, and whole grains each day makes it unnecessary to count grams of fiber or to keep track of how much you are eating of each type of fiber.

Recommendations for Fiber Intake

1. Consume 25 to 35 g of fiber if under age 50, and 20 to 30 g of fiber if over age 50. Most people get less than 15 g of fiber daily.

2. Eat whole grains and vegetables for insoluble fiber. Refined grain products—white bread, white flour, white rice, and pasta—are not good sources of fiber. To get insoluble fiber, you must consume the bran (the outer coating of the grain) that is removed in the processing of many grains, especially wheat milled for flour. Good sources of insoluble fiber include whole-grain cereals, whole-wheat bread, whole-wheat crackers, bulgur, and wheat berries. Vegetables such as broccoli and potatoes with their skins also are good sources of insoluble fiber.

3. Eat oats, barley, legumes, and fruits for soluble fiber.

4. Increase fiber intake gradually over several weeks. A sudden increase of fiber in the diet may cause uncomfortable gas pains.

5. Drink enough water. Insoluble fiber needs fluid to be effective. The standard advice to drink at least eight 8-oz. glasses of water or other fluids every day is being reevaluated, but you should certainly drink whenever you are thirsty.

6. Do not go overboard on fiber. A very high intake can interfere with the absorption of some vitamins and minerals.

VITAMINS AND MINERALS

Vitamins and minerals are essential for virtually all of the biochemical processes necessary for life. They are needed to produce energy, fight disease, and repair injured tissue. One of their most important functions is the activation of enzymes to initiate and control chemical reactions in the body.

The 13 essential vitamins are divided into two major groups: water soluble (vitamin C and the B vitamins) and fat soluble (vitamins A, D, E, and K). With the exception of vitamin B_{12}, water-soluble vitamins cannot be stored in the body and need to be replaced frequently. Fat-soluble vitamins, which can be stored, require less frequent replacement. Important minerals include calcium, magnesium, and potassium.

While true vitamin and mineral deficiencies are rare in developed countries, less-than-optimal intake of certain nutrients is common among Americans. A diminished intake of vitamins and minerals may raise the risk of chronic disease, including cardiovascular disease, colon and breast cancer, bone fractures, as well as pregnancies resulting in neural tube defects.

Multivitamins

Because studies suggest that the diets of most American adults fall short in ideal amounts of vitamins and minerals, a 2002 report in the *Journal of the American Medical Association* advises all adults to consume a daily multivitamin supplement. The recommendation is based on accumulated evidence from more than 100 research studies. Taking a multivitamin supplement can help to fill nutritional gaps in the typical American diet, although the practice is no substitute for eating a balanced diet rich in unprocessed whole foods, which are naturally full of thousands of potentially bioactive substances.

Most multivitamin supplements contain the RDA of all the essential vitamins, except biotin and vitamin K, which are easy to obtain from foods. The supplements also contain a smattering of key minerals. Most men and nonmenstruating women are advised to select a multivitamin supplement that contains little or no iron. Products formulated especially for seniors, however, typically contain less iron and vitamin A, and more calcium, vitamin B_{12}, and vitamin B_6.

While optimal multivitamin doses are beneficial for everyone, high doses of some nutrients, particularly fat-soluble vitamins, are dangerous. A notable example of this is the toxic effect of excessive amounts of vitamin A. Consumers are advised to take multivitamin supplements that contain no more than 5,000 IU of vitamin A; at least 20% should be in the form of beta-carotene. Avoid separate vitamin A supplements, such as cod liver oil.

Taking a supplement in addition to a multivitamin may benefit certain individuals. For example, the elderly are advised to take extra supplements of calcium and vitamin D, as well as a vitamin B_{12} supplement. Women of childbearing age are advised to consume an additional supplement of 400 micrograms (mcg) of folic acid per day.

Everyone is advised to consume a multivitamin with food because nutrients are absorbed best together. In addition, to avoid the expense of name-brand vitamins, experts recommend buying

Vitamins: Sources, Actions, and Benefits

This chart describes and provides sources for the 13 vitamins. In addition, it enumerates the adult Recommended Dietary Allowance (RDA) established by the National Academy of Sciences. For some vitamins, not enough is known to recommend a specific amount; in these cases, the Academy has recommended a range called the Estimated Safe and Adequate Daily Dietary Intake (ESADDI).

Vitamin/Food Sources	What It Does/Potential Benefits	Recommended Intake
Vitamin A. Liver, eggs, fortified milk, fish, fruits and vegetables that contain beta-carotene, such as carrots, sweet potatoes, cantaloupe, leafy greens, tomatoes, apricots, winter squash, red bell peppers, broccoli, and mangoes.	Essential for night vision; helps form and maintain healthy skin and mucous membranes. Beta-carotene is converted in the body to vitamin A; beta-carotene (and other carotenoids) from foods may protect against some cancers and increase resistance to infection in children.	*700 mcg for women; 900 mcg for men.* Vitamin A may be toxic in high doses (over 3,000 mcg), so supplements are not recommended. Beta-carotene supplements may increase lung cancer risk in smokers. In contrast to vitamin A, beta-carotene in food is never toxic.
Vitamin C (ascorbic acid). Citrus fruits and juices, strawberries, peppers, broccoli, potatoes, kale, cauliflower, cantaloupe.	Promotes healthy gums and teeth; aids in iron absorption; maintains normal connective tissue; helps in wound healing. As an antioxidant, it combats adverse effects of free radicals. May reduce the risk of certain cancers.	*75 mg for women; 90 mg for men.* For supplementation, smokers should add 35 mg a day. Tissue levels are not increased further when supplements exceed 250 mg.
Vitamin D. Milk, fish oil, fortified margarine; also produced by the body in response to sunlight.	Promotes strong bones and teeth by aiding absorption of calcium. Helps maintain blood levels of calcium and phosphorus. May reduce the risk of osteoporosis.	*200 IU for adults age 19 to 50; 400 IU for adults age 51 to 70; 600 IU for adults age 70+.* The limited amount of vitamin D in food often makes it necessary to take a supplement.
Vitamin E. Nuts, vegetable oils, margarine, wheat germ, leafy greens, seeds, almonds, olives, whole grains.	As an antioxidant, it combats adverse effects of free radicals. Consult your doctor before using vitamin E supplements if you are taking aspirin or warfarin.	*15 mg.*
Vitamin K. Cauliflower, broccoli, leafy greens, cabbage, milk, soybeans, eggs. Bacteria in the intestine produce most of the vitamin K needed each day.	Essential for normal blood clotting.	*90 mcg for women; 120 mcg for men.* No supplementation necessary or recommended.
Thiamin (B_1). Whole grains, dried beans, lean meats, liver, wheat germ, nuts, brewer's yeast.	Required for the conversion of carbohydrates into energy; necessary for normal function of the brain, nerves, and heart.	*1.1 mg for women; 1.2 mg for men.* No supplementation necessary or recommended.

Vitamin/Food Sources	What It Does/Potential Benefits	Recommended Intake
Riboflavin (B_2). Dairy products, liver, meat, chicken, fish, leafy greens, beans, nuts, eggs.	Helps cells convert carbohydrates into energy; essential for growth, production of red blood cells, and health of skin and eyes.	*1.1 mg for women; 1.3 mg for men.* No supplementation necessary or recommended.
Niacin (B_3). Nuts, grains, meat, fish, chicken, liver, dairy products.	Aids in release of energy from foods; helps maintain healthy skin, nerves, and digestive system. Large doses may be prescribed by a doctor to lower low density lipoprotein (LDL) cholesterol and triglyceride levels and raise high density lipoprotein (HDL) cholesterol levels.	*14 mg for women; 16 mg for men.* When used in large doses to lower cholesterol, may cause flushing, nausea, gout, liver damage, and increased blood glucose levels. Do not exceed 35 mg/day unless prescribed by a doctor.
Vitamin B_6 (pyridoxine). Whole grains, bananas, meat, beans, nuts, wheat germ, chicken, fish, liver.	Important in chemical reactions of proteins and amino acids; helps maintain brain function and form red blood cells. May boost immunity in the elderly. May lower homocysteine levels, high levels of which may increase risk of coronary heart disease (CHD).	*1.5 mg for women age 51+; 1.7 mg for men age 51+.* Megadoses can cause numbness and other neurological disorders.
Folate (B_9) (folic acid, folacin). Leafy greens, wheat germ, liver, beans, whole and fortified grains, broccoli, citrus fruit.	Important in the synthesis of DNA, in normal growth, and in protein metabolism. Adequate intake reduces risk of certain birth defects. May protect against CHD by lowering homocysteine levels.	*400 mcg.* Can be derived from both fortified foods and supplements. Doses should not exceed 1,000 mcg/day.
Vitamin B_{12} (cobalamin). Liver, beef, pork, poultry, eggs, dairy products, seafood, fortified cereals.	Necessary for production of red blood cells; maintains normal functioning of nervous system.	*2.4 mcg.* Strict vegetarians may need supplements. Despite claims, no benefits from megadoses.
Pantothenic acid. Whole grains, dried beans, eggs, milk, liver.	Vital for metabolism of food and production of essential body chemicals.	*5 mg.* No supplementation necessary or recommended.
Biotin. Eggs, milk, liver, brewer's yeast, mushrooms, bananas, grains.	Important in metabolism of protein, carbohydrates, and fats.	*30 mcg.* No supplementation necessary or recommended.

inexpensive, generic-brand multivitamins sold at pharmacies or discount shops.

B VITAMINS: FOLIC ACID, VITAMIN B_6, AND VITAMIN B_{12}

B vitamins are vital for the breakdown and utilization of carbohydrates, fats, and proteins, and they also help to ensure the proper functioning of the nervous system and the synthesis of red blood cells and genetic material. Folic acid is essential during the early months of pregnancy to prevent birth defects, such as spina bifida and cleft palate.

Older adults may have greater requirements for certain B vitamins, particularly vitamins B_6 and B_{12}. A lack of vitamin B_{12} can cause a form of dementia in older people that may be mistaken for Alzheimer's disease. An insufficient intake of vitamin B_6 may impair immune function in older adults, and the absorption of vitamin B_{12} diminishes with age. Some experts estimate that 10% to 30% of older adults are unable to absorb vitamin B_{12} efficiently from food, owing to alterations in the cells lining the digestive tract or diminished secretion of a substance called intrinsic factor that is needed to absorb vitamin B_{12}. Experts believe that most older adults can benefit from taking a daily B_{12} supplement in addition to a multivitamin to ensure adequate intake of B vitamins.

B Vitamins and Heart Disease

Vitamin B_6, vitamin B_{12}, and especially folic acid may be important for the prevention of cardiovascular disease. They affect blood levels of the amino acid homocysteine by regulating its formation and conversion to other amino acids. It has been known for 30 years that people with a condition called homocystinuria—an inherited metabolic defect that results in extremely high blood levels of homocysteine—develop premature atherosclerosis and often suffer a heart attack or stroke before age 30. Now, researchers have found that people with far more moderate homocysteine elevations are at increased risk for cardiovascular disease.

Just how excess homocysteine contributes to arterial disease is not known. Some animal studies suggest that homocysteine damages the cells lining blood vessels and paves the way for the buildup of plaque. Other research suggests that homocysteine increases the formation of blood clots, which can obstruct an artery and cause a heart attack or stroke.

There is no doubt that folic acid and homocysteine levels in the blood are inversely related—that is, when folic acid levels are higher, homocysteine levels are lower. Many studies have clearly shown that folic acid supplements lower homocysteine levels. It is not yet clear whether increasing folic acid intake, alone or in combination with vitamin B_6, can lower the risk of arterial disease, but much of the evidence points in that direction. More research needs to be done to determine whether an adequate intake of folic acid and vitamin B_6 can reduce the risk of arterial disease.

Recommendations for Intake of B Vitamins

1. Get plenty of folic acid every day. The Recommended Dietary Allowance (RDA) for this vitamin is 400 mcg. Good sources include enriched breads and cereals, dried peas and beans, oranges, orange juice, green vegetables, and whole grains.

2. Eat foods rich in vitamin B_6. Meeting the RDA of 1.3 mg (for women) to 1.7 mg (for men) is all that is necessary. Good sources of vitamin B_6 include fish, meats, poultry, avocados, and bananas.

3. Maintain an adequate vitamin B_{12} intake. The RDA for people over 50 is 2.4 mcg per day. People age 50 and older can meet the RDA mainly by consuming foods fortified with B_{12} or with a supplement containing B_{12}. On the other hand, vegetarians who eat no animal products (B_{12} is found only in meat, poultry, shellfish, fish, eggs, and dairy products) need to take a vitamin B_{12} supplement. Vitamin B_6 and iron enhance vitamin B_{12} absorption. People taking supplements of folic acid should also add 1 mcg of vitamin B_{12} daily.

4. Take a multivitamin. People with elevated levels of homocysteine should consider a multivitamin, which will supply all of the above B vitamins. Most multivitamins contain the amounts recommended above.

CALCIUM AND VITAMIN D

Most people are aware that calcium is essential for the formation and strength of bones, but few people realize that it fulfills other important functions. For example, calcium in the bloodstream is involved in blood clotting, blood pressure control, enzyme activation, contraction and relaxation of muscles (including the heart), nerve transmission, and membrane permeability (controlling the passage of fluids and other substances in and out of cells).

Along with calcium, you also need vitamin D to maintain the body's calcium stores. Without vitamin D, ingested calcium is

NEW RESEARCH

Low Childhood Milk Intake Increases Fracture Risk in Adults

A low intake of milk during childhood and adolescence may contribute to reduced bone loss and a greater risk of osteoporotic fractures later in life.

A recent study of 3,251 non-Hispanic white women found that women age 20 to 49 who consumed less than one glass of milk a day during childhood (age 5 to 12) had a hip bone mass that was 5.6% lower than that in women who drank at least one glass of milk a day. Low milk intake in adolescence (age 13 to 17) was associated with a 3% reduction in bone mass at the hip.

Also, women age 50 and older who had a low childhood milk intake had a two times greater risk of fracture compared with women who consumed one or more glasses of milk daily. The authors estimate that low milk intake during childhood may be responsible for about 11% of osteoporotic fractures in women age 50 and older.

According to an accompanying editorial, the investigators might have found an even stronger association between milk intake and risk of fractures later in life if they had accounted for each glass of milk over one per day that the women drank in childhood and adolescence, instead of grouping all women who drank one or more glasses daily into a single category.

AMERICAN JOURNAL OF CLINICAL NUTRITION
Volume 77, pages 10 and 257
January 2003

Are You Getting Enough Vitamin D?

Deficiencies of this important vitamin—which has been linked to myriad health benefits—may be widespread.

Called the sunshine vitamin, vitamin D is made in our skin upon exposure to small amounts of bright sunlight. Vital for well-being, vitamin D is best known for its important role in bone health. By enhancing calcium absorption and maintaining healthy levels of phosphorous, vitamin D is essential for building and preserving well-formed, sturdy bones. Along with its activity in the skeleton, vitamin D helps to ensure that the brain, heart, pancreas, skin, stomach, and reproductive organs are working properly. In addition, vitamin D helps a variety of cells to mature, including infection-fighting cells of the immune system.

Getting Enough

Getting enough vitamin D is easy if you regularly spend some time outdoors: Sunlight provides at least 90% of the vitamin D that we need. For adequate vitamin D formation, skin must be exposed to the sun for a short amount of time (15 minutes per day) without sunscreen; wearing a sunscreen with a sun protection factor (SPF) of 8 or higher blocks almost 98% of the sun's rays.

In the absence of enough sunshine, the body can obtain vitamin D through the diet and supplementation. Recommended daily intakes of vitamin D are set at 200 international units (IU) for people 19 to 50, 400 IU for people 51 to 70, and 600 IU for people over age 70, although some experts think daily vitamin D requirements should be more. Dietary requirements increase with age because the skin's ability to make vitamin D diminishes with age. Though few foods are plentiful in vitamin D, the top sources are fatty fish such as mackerel, salmon, and sardines. Other types of seafood, as well as fortified cereals, dairy foods, and soy foods, offer appreciable amounts of vitamin D.

Vitamin D Deficiencies

Despite the ease with which our skin makes vitamin D, recent evidence suggests that deficiencies are far more common than previously thought. Concern about skin cancer, a sedentary indoor lifestyle, and a poor diet may account for some of the deficiencies. Older and housebound adults are at particularly high risk. In one study of 98 postmenopausal women admitted to a Boston hospital with hip fractures, half of the women were found to be deficient in vitamin D. Another investigation of 290 hospital inpatients showed that 57% were deficient in vitamin D, and 22% were deemed severely deficient.

Surprisingly, vitamin D deficiencies may also be prevalent among healthy, young adults in the United States, particularly during the winter when sun exposure is low, and throughout the year in people with dark skin, which slows vitamin D formation. In a 2002 survey, one third of 138 active adults age 18 to 29 in Boston were deficient in vitamin D by the end of the winter. Another recent study of approximately 3,000 American women age 15 to 49 found inadequate circulating levels of vitamin D in 4% of white women and 41% of black women.

Lasting Effects of Deficiencies

Mounting evidence suggests that the widespread vitamin D deficiencies may lead to serious and lasting health consequences, especially bone loss. The most severe vitamin D deficiencies are marked by soft, bent,

poorly absorbed from the intestines. In addition, vitamin D strengthens the immune system. Although vitamin D is found naturally in only a few foods, the body can usually produce enough in response to sunlight. (For more information on getting enough vitamin D, see the feature above.)

Calcium, Vitamin D, and Osteoporosis

An adequate intake of calcium protects against the development of osteoporosis, which causes bones to become porous, brittle, and susceptible to fractures. According to the National Osteoporosis Foundation, approximately 10 million Americans—80%

Under Investigation

Very preliminary research has found possible links between vitamin D deficiencies and a number of serious health consequences, including high blood pressure, cancer, and autoimmune diseases.

High blood pressure. Low levels of vitamin D have been linked to high blood pressure. Preliminary studies suggest that blacks who are chronically low in vitamin D are more likely to suffer from high blood pressure.

Cancer. Population studies have found that people who live in less sunny climates (at higher latitudes) have the greatest chance of dying of cancers of the breast, colon, and prostate. In fact, the risk of dying of these cancers is twice as high in the northeastern United States than in southwestern regions, regardless of any differences in diet.

A number of studies have specifically linked low vitamin D levels to cancer. In one study of over 100 adults, those with low levels of circulating vitamin D were 50% more likely to develop colon cancer than participants with normal vitamin D levels. Another four-year investigation of over 120,000 healthy adults found that men who consumed diets sufficient in vitamin D had a significantly reduced risk of developing colon cancer.

Autoimmune diseases. Laboratory findings indicate that vitamin D influences certain key activities of immune cells. For instance, vitamin D helps infection-fighting cells of the immune system to mature. Furthermore, studies have shown that people who live in less sunny climates (farther from the equator) are more likely to develop common autoimmune diseases, such as arthritis, multiple sclerosis, and type 1 diabetes. In Finland, for example, annual sunlight is very low and the risk of type 1 diabetes is the highest in the world. One study of 10,000 children in northern Finland found that those who regularly received a supplement of vitamin D were significantly less likely to develop type 1 diabetes during the first year of life.

fragile bones. In children, this condition is known as rickets. In adults, the disorder is called osteomalacia and may be accompanied by bone and muscle pain as well as muscle weakness—symptoms that are at times misdiagnosed as fibromyalgia.

Low levels of vitamin D also contribute to osteoporosis and may raise the risk of fractures. Consuming a supplement of both vitamin D and calcium prevents loss of bone mineral density and lessens destructive bone turnover.

Supplements Can Help

A daily multivitamin supplement can help to meet vitamin D requirements when diet and sun exposure are inadequate. In one study of 165 active adults, participants who did not regularly take a daily multivitamin supplement were three times more likely to have a vitamin D deficiency than those who consumed a daily multivitamin. Concentrated supplements, such as cod liver oil, are not recommended because their vitamin D content is so large that they can cause adverse effects. When consumed in excess, vitamin D is the most toxic of all of the vitamins; it can lead to mental changes, nausea, vomiting, heart abnormalities, kidney stones, and even death. It can also lead to high blood calcium levels (hypercalcemia), which may cause fatigue, muscle weakness, confusion, drowsiness, and coma. To prevent toxicity, the upper daily limit of vitamin D is fixed at 1,000 IU for infants and 2,000 IU for everyone over the age of one.

of them women—suffer from osteoporosis. An additional 18 million have low bone mineral density, which is a risk factor for osteoporosis. While postmenopausal women are at highest risk, men also are susceptible to osteoporosis, particularly when they reach age 65.

When blood levels of calcium are too low, calcium can be released from bones, which contain 99% of body calcium. Bones are constantly broken down and rebuilt throughout life. This bone turnover becomes a problem only when calcium use outpaces calcium intake, because the body will then sacrifice bone in order to maintain blood calcium levels needed for these other crucial functions. Over time, a deficit in dietary calcium can result in osteoporosis.

Calcium, Vitamin D, and Other Disorders

Calcium may offer a small reduction of blood pressure in people with high blood pressure, and vitamin D may help people with osteoarthritis. Both calcium and vitamin D appear to have a modest protective effect against colon cancer.

Recommendations for Calcium and Vitamin D Intake

1. If you are between the ages of 19 and 50, try to get 1,000 mg of calcium a day. This level of calcium intake helps to maintain calcium stores in bones.

2. At age 51, increase calcium intake to 1,200 mg per day. To build peak bone mass and prevent osteoporosis, however, men and postmenopausal women over age 65 require 1,500 mg of calcium daily as well as an intake of vitamin D ranging from 400 to 600 IU a day.

3. Try to get as much calcium as possible through your diet. Milk and other dairy products are the most concentrated sources. However, use only fat-free or low-fat dairy products; not only is their reduced saturated fat content a benefit, but they are also slightly higher in calcium than full-fat dairy products.

While dairy products are the principal source of dietary calcium, people with lactose intolerance and those who prefer not to consume dairy foods can benefit from nondairy dietary sources of calcium. For example, nondairy calcium can be found in some brands of calcium-fortified juice, canned salmon and sardines with the bones (the bones are soft and edible), firm tofu (make sure the label says the tofu has been processed with calcium), white beans, as well as soybeans, bok choy, and broccoli. Though spinach contains some calcium, it is also rich in oxalates, which interfere with calcium absorption.

4. Do not hesitate to use supplements to make up for calcium shortfalls. Although food is the best source of calcium, if you are unable to meet your calcium requirement through diet alone, a supplement can help you reach your daily calcium needs. Determine how much calcium you get in your diet, and use supplements to meet the recommended intakes, not to exceed them. Up to 2,500 mg of calcium a day is considered safe for adults.

Getting calcium from milk is pretty straightforward. If you drink a glass of milk, you will be getting about 300 mg of so-called ele-

NEW RESEARCH

Vitamin D May Prevent Hip Fractures Better than Calcium

Although the prevention of hip fractures has focused on calcium intake, vitamin D may be more important.

Women in a new observational study who consumed 12.5 micrograms (mcg) or more of vitamin D daily (from food or supplements) were 37% less likely to have a hip fracture than those who consumed less than 3.5 mcg daily. By contrast, women with high calcium intakes (1,200 mg per day or more) were just as likely to have a hip fracture as those with low intakes (less than 600 mg daily). Also, higher milk intake did not lower the risk of hip fracture. The study included 72,337 postmenopausal women who were followed for 18 years with periodic dietary assessments.

Randomized trials of calcium supplementation have shown that calcium intake can increase bone mass and decrease fracture risk in postmenopausal women. However, calcium was often given with vitamin D in these trials, clouding the issue of which nutrient is more important for bone health. Although milk is a common source of vitamin D, milk also contains vitamin A, which can have a detrimental effect on bone.

Postmenopausal women can improve their vitamin D intake through more frequent consumption of fatty fish such as salmon and sardines or the use of supplements, the authors conclude.

AMERICAN JOURNAL OF CLINICAL NUTRITION
Volume 77, page 504
February 2003

mental calcium. (All calcium guidelines refer to elemental calcium.) However, in supplement form elemental calcium must be combined with a weak acid to form a chemical compound. The different types of calcium compounds include calcium carbonate, calcium phosphate, and calcium citrate, each of which contains a different amount of elemental calcium (this is the amount of calcium that is listed on the label).

Calcium carbonate and calcium citrate contain the highest percentage of elemental calcium per tablet—40% and 30%, respectively. Studies show that the calcium in citrate-based supplements is more efficiently absorbed than the calcium in carbonate-based ones. Calcium carbonate pills should be taken with meals because calcium absorption from such tablets is improved by the presence of gastric acid. Because calcium supplements are available in a wide range of preparations and strengths, selecting the right one can be complicated.

Calcium supplements (as well as dietary calcium) are best absorbed when taken (or consumed) several times a day in amounts of 500 mg or less. Ask your physician to help you determine which type of calcium supplement is best for you.

5. Take calcium supplements with meals. Do not take supplements at bedtime, when the acid content of the stomach is low. Many older people do not produce enough stomach acid between meals to dissolve calcium tablets thoroughly.

6. Expose your skin to sunlight to generate vitamin D production. The recommended intake for vitamin D is 400 IU per day for men and women age 51 to 70, and 600 IU for those over 70. Exposure to sunlight can generate 200 IU in just 10 minutes if the hands and face are exposed. However, sunscreen with a sun protection factor (SPF) of 8 or higher can block the ultraviolet rays needed to produce vitamin D. Therefore, you should spend 10 to 15 minutes outside prior to applying sunscreen. Older people may need slightly longer exposure to compensate for the decreased ability of their skin to synthesize vitamin D in response to sunlight.

7. If you live in a northern climate, consider taking a multivitamin with vitamin D in the winter. Most multivitamins contain 400 IU of vitamin D. People who are homebound or live in a nursing home need vitamin D supplements throughout the year. All people with osteoporosis or low bone mineral density should take 400 to 800 IU of vitamin D—not as a multivitamin but either alone or in combination with a calcium supplement. Consult your physician to see what type of supplement is best for you.

Minerals: Sources, Actions, and Benefits

As with vitamins, the National Academy of Sciences has established a Recommended Dietary Allowance (RDA) or Estimated Safe and Adequate Daily Dietary Intake (ESADDI) for minerals. The chart below gives a description of each mineral as well as the Academy's recommendation for intake.

Mineral/Food Sources	What It Does	Recommended Intake
Calcium. Milk and milk products, canned salmon and sardines eaten with bones, dark green leafy vegetables, shellfish, some fortified cereals.	Major component of bones and teeth; helps prevent or minimize osteoporosis; helps regulate heartbeat, blood clotting, muscle contraction, and nerve conduction. May help prevent hypertension.	*1,000 mg for adults age 19 to 50; 1,200 mg for adults age 51+.*
Chloride. Table salt, fish.	Helps maintain fluid and acid–base balance; component of gastric juice.	*No RDA.*
Chromium. Meat, cheese, whole grains, brewer's yeast.	Important in metabolism of carbohydrates and fats. Deficiency may impair the action of insulin.	*25 mcg for women age 19 to 50; 20 mcg for women age 51+; 35 mcg for men age 19 to 50; 30 mcg for men age 51+.*
Copper. Shellfish, nuts, beans, seeds, organ meats, whole grains, potatoes.	Formation of red blood cells; helps keep bones, nerves, and immune system healthy.	*900 mcg.*
Fluoride. Fluoridated water and foods grown or cooked in it, marine fish (with bones), tea.	Contributes to solid bone and tooth formation. Reduces dental cavities.	*3 mg for women; 4 mg for men.*
Iodine. Primarily from iodized salt, but also seafood, seaweed food products, vegetables grown in iodine-rich areas. Widely dispersed in the food supply.	Necessary for the formation of thyroid hormone and thus for normal cell metabolism; prevents goiter (enlargement of the thyroid).	*150 mcg.*
Iron. Liver, kidneys, red meats, eggs, peas, beans, nuts, dried fruits, green leafy vegetables, enriched grain products, fortified cereals. Cooking in iron pots adds iron, especially to acidic foods.	Essential component of hemoglobin (which carries oxygen in red blood cells) and myoglobin (in muscle); part of several enzymes and proteins in the body. Heme iron, found in animal products, is better absorbed by the body than nonheme iron, found in plants.	*18 mg for women age 19 to 50; 8 mg for women age 51+; 8 mg for men.* There may be a danger in iron supplements for people who do not know they have hemachromatosis.

Mineral/Food Sources	What It Does	Recommended Intake
Magnesium. Wheat bran, whole grains, raw leafy green vegetables, nuts, soybeans, bananas.	Aids in bone growth; aids function of nerves and muscles, including regulation of normal heart rhythm.	*310 mg for women age 19 to 30; 320 mg for women age 31+; 400 mg for men age 19 to 30; 420 mg for men age 31+.*
Manganese. Nuts, whole grains, vegetables, fruits, instant coffee, tea, cocoa powder, beans.	Needed for energy production and reproduction. May also be essential for building bones. Excess may interfere with iron absorption.	*1.8 mg for women; 2.3 mg for men.*
Molybdenum. Peas, beans, cereal grains, organ meats, some dark green vegetables.	Aids in bone growth and strengthening of teeth; important in energy metabolism.	*45 mcg.*
Phosphorus. Meats, poultry, fish, dairy products, eggs, dried peas and beans, soft drinks, nuts; present in almost all foods.	Major component of bones and teeth; present in cell membranes and genetic material. Vital for energy metabolism.	*700 mg.*
Potassium. Most foods, especially oranges and orange juice, bananas, potatoes (with skin), tomatoes, potatoes, greens, dried beans, brussels sprouts, dried fruits, yogurt, meat, poultry, milk.	Vital for muscle contraction, nerve impulses, and function of heart and kidneys. Helps regulate blood pressure and water balance in cells.	*1,600 to 2,000 mg minimum.*
Selenium. Fish, shellfish, red meat, nuts, grains, eggs, chicken, garlic, organ meats; amount in vegetables depends on soil.	Part of enzymes that act as antioxidants to prevent cell damage. Needed for proper immune response.	*55 mcg.* Large doses can be toxic.
Sodium. Table salt, salt added to prepared foods (such as cheese, smoked meats, and fast foods), baking soda.	Helps regulate blood pressure and water balance in the body.	*2,400 mg maximum.*
Zinc. Oysters, crabmeat, liver, eggs, poultry, brewer's yeast, wheat germ, milk, beans.	Important in activity of enzymes for cell division, growth, and repair (wound healing), as well as proper functioning of immune system. Maintains taste and smell acuity.	*8 mg for women; 11 mg for men.*

SODIUM AND POTASSIUM

Sodium, found outside cells, and potassium, found mainly inside cells, are minerals that work together to maintain fluid balance in the body. In addition, they are involved in the regulation of muscle contraction and nerve transmission and play an important role in controlling blood pressure.

Although sodium occurs naturally in foods, the average person consumes most dietary sodium from table salt and other compounds—for example, sodium bicarbonate (baking soda) or monosodium glutamate (MSG)—added to foods in processing, in cooking, or at the table.

Keep in mind when reading the information in this section that sodium and salt are not the same thing. Only 40% of table salt (sodium chloride) is sodium. All of the values in the following refer to amounts of sodium, not salt.

Sodium, Potassium, and Hypertension

Overall, Americans tend to get too much sodium—about 3,900 mg per day, which is nearly twice the recommended amount—and too little potassium. This imbalance may contribute to high blood pressure. Experts continue to debate whether everyone needs to lower sodium intake to prevent or control high blood pressure. While many experts maintain that everyone should cut back on sodium intake, some hold that sodium reduction is worthwhile only when blood pressure is too high or in those who have a family history of high blood pressure.

Part of the debate results from an incomplete understanding of how sodium increases blood pressure. Researchers know that higher sodium levels promote water retention, which in turn increases blood volume and may ultimately lead to higher blood pressure. Excess sodium is usually excreted in the urine, but 30% to 50% of people with hypertension cannot efficiently get rid of excess sodium. Sodium can also constrict small blood vessels, which causes greater resistance to blood flow. How sodium produces blood vessel constriction remains unknown.

High blood pressure is defined as having a systolic blood pressure (the upper number) of 140 mm Hg or higher and/or a diastolic blood pressure (the lower number) of 90 mm Hg or higher. Studies estimate that if everyone stopped adding salt to food (which accounts for about a third of the sodium in most diets), the number of people who need antihypertensive medication would be cut in half.

In 1997, the results from the DASH (Dietary Approaches to Stop Hypertension) trial proved that diet could reduce blood pressure. The diet used in the eight-week study consisted of 8 to 10 servings of fruits and vegetables and 2 to 3 servings of low-fat dairy products each day. The diet also promoted plant sources of protein at least once or twice a week. By the end of the trial, the DASH diet had reduced blood pressure by an average of 5.5/3 mm Hg compared with the control diet. While the DASH diet is highly effective for prevention of hypertension, some of the most impressive results were in people who already had hypertension. These individuals, who had blood pressures of 140/90 mm Hg or greater, lowered their levels by 11/5.5 mm Hg, which is as low as (or lower than) the results produced by a single antihypertensive medication.

Results from a subsequent study, the DASH-Sodium trial, published in *The New England Journal of Medicine* in 2001 indicate that combining the DASH diet with a reduced sodium intake can lower blood pressure more than either measure alone. In the trial, participants followed a diet that combined the DASH diet with one of three levels of sodium intake (3,300 mg, 2,400 mg, or 1,500 mg per day). Those participants with hypertension who consumed the least sodium had a systolic blood pressure that was almost 12 mm Hg lower than that of people who ate the typical American diet with a high sodium level.

A large part of the success of the DASH-Sodium diet may be its high potassium content of about 4,400 mg daily (roughly the amount in 11 bananas). Research indicates that potassium lowers blood pressure by relaxing arteries. But the interplay of all essential nutrients in the diet, as well as fiber, is probably just as important as any single vitamin or mineral.

The DASH diet may also help to improve cholesterol levels. According to a study in the *American Journal of Clinical Nutrition*, the diet reduces total cholesterol an average of 13.7 mg/dL and LDL cholesterol an average of 10.7 mg/dL. In another recent study, the diet reduced total cholesterol an average of 13.7 mg/dL and LDL cholesterol an average of 10.7 mg/dL.

Sodium and Other Disorders

There are several other reasons to reduce sodium in your diet. A high-sodium diet can increase the loss of calcium in the urine, which in turn triggers removal of calcium from bones. A very high intake of sodium (3,000 mg or more daily) can also raise the risk of stomach cancer because sodium irritates the lining of the stomach,

NEW RESEARCH

Eating Fruit May Reduce the Risk of Stroke

Fruits and vegetables may offer some protection against an ischemic stroke, according to a recent study. (An ischemic stroke, the most common type, is caused by a blockage in a blood vessel in or leading to the brain.)

Researchers in Denmark assessed the dietary habits of more than 54,000 men and women (age 50 to 64) between 1993 and 1997. Approximately three years later, 266 participants had experienced an ischemic stroke.

After adjusting for other stroke risk factors such as blood pressure, smoking history, and total calorie intake, people with the highest intake of fruits and vegetables (an average of 22 oz. per day) were 28% less likely to have an ischemic stroke than people with the lowest intake (an average of less than 5 oz. per day). The association was strongest for fruit: People who ate the most fruit were 40% less likely to have an ischemic stroke than people who ate the least.

When the data on individual fruits and vegetables were examined, citrus fruits were linked with the greatest reduction in stroke risk, while mushrooms, onions, garlic, and stalk vegetables (such as asparagus) were not associated with a reduction in risk. Low potassium intake has been linked with increasing stroke risk, and fruits (especially bananas) tend to be high in potassium.

AMERICAN JOURNAL OF CLINICAL NUTRITION
Volume 78, page 57
July 2003

especially in people who have had ulcers. Finally, excess sodium contributes to kidney disease as an extension of its effect on hypertension. Chronic high blood pressure damages organs by injuring the blood vessels that supply them, and the kidneys are particularly vulnerable to this effect.

Recommendations for Sodium and Potassium Intake

1. Don't add salt to foods. One teaspoon of salt contains 2,130 mg of sodium. At first, a low-sodium diet may make food taste bland, but within six to eight weeks your palate will adjust, and the amount of salt you once used will make foods taste too salty.

2. If you have hypertension, do not consume more than 2,000 mg of sodium daily. Those individuals who have a particular sensitivity to sodium should consume even less.

3. Flavor foods with herbs, spices, and citrus juices. These seasonings can help perk up foods and compensate for the flavor lost from the reduction in salt.

4. Read food labels carefully for sodium content. Packaged and processed foods supply about two thirds of the sodium in the average diet. Minimize your use of high-sodium products, such as luncheon meats, sausages, smoked meats and fish, hot dogs, canned shellfish, canned soups, frozen dinners, condiments (relish, mustard, ketchup, soy sauce, and pickles), cheese, and processed snack foods.

5. Remember that sodium comes in many forms, not just salt. Baking soda, monosodium glutamate (MSG), onion salt, garlic salt, and some other flavorings also are sources of sodium.

6. Try salt alternatives. Salt alternatives—such as Cardia and Morton's Lite Salt, which contain about half the sodium of table salt—can be an option for some people. However, people with kidney problems and those taking potassium-sparing diuretics for hypertension or heart failure should not use these products because they contain more potassium than regular salt. Speak with your doctor first before using these salt alternatives.

7. Look for reduced-sodium packaged foods. Sodium claims made on labels must meet certain standards: Low-sodium foods have 140 mg or less per serving, very low sodium means 35 mg or less, and sodium free has 5 mg or less. Unsalted or no-salt-added foods generally contain only naturally occurring sodium.

8. Get about 2,000 mg of potassium a day. Eat more fruits, vegetables, legumes, and grains. Bananas, kidney beans, lentils, oranges, orange juice, yogurt, cantaloupe, prunes, and potatoes are just a few of the foods that are high in potassium—and low in sodium as well.

ALCOHOL

The role of alcohol in a healthy diet is confusing. While moderate alcohol consumption has some undeniable health benefits, alcohol also adds extra calories, interferes with the action of many medications, and when consumed in excess over a long period of time, can cause some types of heart disease and raise blood pressure. Fatty liver and cirrhosis are major consequences of alcohol abuse. In addition, alcohol is a leading cause of car accidents.

Studies in both men and women have shown that having one to two alcoholic drinks per day is associated with a 30% to 60% reduction in the risk of developing CHD, and also helps protect against ischemic stroke (the type caused by a blood clot in an atherosclerotic carotid or cerebral artery). Just how alcohol prevents CHD and strokes is a subject of much scientific debate, but it is generally accepted that about half of the risk reduction comes from an increase in HDL cholesterol levels. The rest of the protection may be due to alcohol's ability to reduce clot formation in the coronary and cerebral arteries.

For women, however, there is a downside to moderate drinking. Daily consumption of even small amounts of alcohol appears to increase the chances of breast cancer. Studies have shown a 30% to 60% rise in breast cancer risk for women who have one or two alcoholic drinks per day. The risk increases steeply—some studies show it more than doubles—as alcohol consumption rises to three or more drinks per day. Recent alcohol consumption appears to have a greater impact on risk than alcohol consumption early in life.

A report from the Iowa Women's Health Study, involving over 41,000 women, found that the effect of alcohol on breast cancer risk was limited to women taking estrogen replacement therapy (ERT). This result was not confirmed by other studies; however, one study found that in postmenopausal women on ERT, drinking alcohol tripled blood levels of estradiol, a form of estrogen, and estrogen has been shown to promote breast cancer. The researchers who conducted this study speculated that the combination of ERT and alcohol may increase the risk of breast cancer more than either one alone.

Recommendations for Alcohol Consumption

1. If you don't currently drink alcohol, don't start. Experts do not recommend that teetotalers begin drinking alcohol, but instead should take other steps to reduce their risk of CHD.

2. Men who drink should limit themselves to one to two alcoholic drinks per day. This amount of alcohol is enough to reduce CHD risk. However, it may impact the ability to drive and operate other machinery. (A drink is defined as 12 oz. of beer, 5 oz. of wine, or 1½ oz. of 80-proof spirits.)

3. Women who drink but have no CHD risk factors should limit alcohol to fewer than seven drinks per week. Having a few drinks per week probably does not increase the odds of getting breast cancer, but it is not known whether this amount of alcohol can prevent CHD.

4. Women who drink and have CHD (or an increased risk of CHD) should have no more than one drink per day. For a woman at risk for CHD, the benefits of moderate alcohol consumption may outweigh the risks. However, keep in mind that there are many ways to reduce CHD risk but few known ways to reduce the risk of breast cancer.

5. The type of alcoholic drink does not matter. Some studies have emphasized the protective effect of red wine in reducing CHD risk, but most experts agree that wine (red or white), beer, or spirits all have the same effect.

6. Remember that heavy alcohol consumption is a health risk. Heavy drinking (more than two alcoholic drinks per day) can cause a variety of life-threatening diseases, including hypertension, stroke, cardiomyopathy (an enlargement of the heart), and cirrhosis.

7. Certain people should avoid alcohol altogether. They include people with hypertriglyceridemia, pancreatitis, liver disease, porphyria, uncontrolled hypertension, and heart failure. Anyone with a past or current problem with alcohol should not drink. And of course, anyone who will be driving should abstain from alcohol.

ANTIOXIDANTS

Antioxidants are substances that help to counteract cell damage resulting from the formation of free radicals during normal metabolism. Free radicals are molecules that are highly reactive because they are missing one or more electrons. They seek to combine with other molecules, and can set off a chain reaction that rapidly passes electrons from molecule to molecule. At times, this process can be beneficial: For example, free radicals help the body fight bacteria and viruses. However, the rapid exchange of electrons can also damage cell membranes and DNA. Excess free radical production is now thought to contribute to many diseases, including CHD, cancer, and cataracts.

A variety of antioxidants can either neutralize free radicals or repair the damage caused by them. Health problems can arise, however, when the body's production of free radicals overwhelms its natural antioxidant defenses. Foods that contain antioxidants—such as vitamins C and E, the mineral selenium, and a collection of plant pigments known as carotenoids (which includes beta-carotene)—can add to the body's supply of antioxidants. Other substances found in plants, known collectively as phytochemicals (see the section on phytochemicals, page 41), may also act as antioxidants. Each antioxidant has a different mode of action, and many of them appear to work together. For example, vitamin C helps to regenerate vitamin E once it has become oxidized. Therefore, it is important that your diet supply adequate amounts of all of the antioxidants to achieve this synergy.

Antioxidants and CHD

Numerous studies have shown that people who eat a lot of fruits and vegetables are less likely to develop CHD. Some researchers attribute this benefit to the antioxidants in these foods, especially vitamin C, vitamin E, beta-carotene, and other carotenoids. In studies that measured blood levels of these nutrients, high levels were associated with a reduced risk of CHD.

However, three large trials have shown that vitamin E supplements provided no benefits in patients with known CHD. A major report recently issued by the Food and Nutrition Board of the National Academy of Sciences—the main authority in the United States for nutritional recommendations—also concluded that vitamin E in supplement form serves no purpose in helping to reduce CHD. And a study in *The New England Journal of Medicine* found that taking antioxidant supplements containing vitamins E and C, beta-carotene, and selenium did not reduce heart attacks in patients with established heart disease, normal LDL cholesterol, and low HDL cholesterol. Drug therapy with simvastatin (Zocor) and niacin produced marked improvements in HDL cholesterol levels, arterial narrowing, and heart attack risk. But combining the drug therapy with antioxidants lessened these benefits.

Moreover, antioxidant supplementation may blunt the benefits of cholesterol drugs, suggests a study in *Arteriosclerosis, Thrombosis, and Vascular Biology*. Researchers treated 153 coronary artery disease patients with drug therapy (a statin with niacin) alone, drug therapy with antioxidants (vitamins E and C, beta-carotene, and selenium), antioxidants alone, or placebo. Cholesterol levels improved more in patients on drug therapy alone. The improvement

NEW RESEARCH

Mediterranean Diet Healthful

Eating a traditional Mediterranean diet appears to decrease the overall risk of premature death, as well as risks posed by coronary heart disease (CHD) and cancer. This recent finding supports previous research asserting that the diet confers health benefits.

Interviewers questioned over 22,000 adult Greeks about their diets. Respondents reported how frequently they ate various food items and the size of a typical portion. They were then tracked for up to eight years. A traditional Mediterranean diet, which many Greeks follow, is characterized by a high intake of plant foods (whole grains, vegetables, legumes, fruits, and nuts); moderate consumption of poultry, fish, and wine; olive oil as the main added fat; and a low intake of saturated fats, such as red meat and full-fat dairy.

The more closely people adhered to the Mediterranean diet, the lower their risk of dying of CHD, cancer, or any cause during follow-up. There were no links between individual food groups and mortality.

Although this study cannot completely rule out the possibility that the benefit of the Mediterranean diet was the result of coexisting healthy lifestyle habits, the investigators did control for a number of these. This study adds support for diets high in plant foods and low in saturated fat.

THE NEW ENGLAND JOURNAL OF MEDICINE
Volume 348, page 2599
June 26, 2003

produced by drug therapy with antioxidants was similar to that of placebo. Make sure to check with your doctor before taking extra vitamin E if you are taking daily blood-thinning medications such as warfarin (Coumadin) or aspirin, because vitamin E also reduces the ability of the blood to clot.

Antioxidants and Cancer

Adequate intakes of beta-carotene and vitamin C have been linked to a reduced risk of cancers of the esophagus, stomach, pancreas, lung, colon, rectum, prostate, breast, ovaries, and cervix. Several studies found that people with low intakes or blood levels of antioxidants have a higher risk of these cancers.

In the studies that showed protective effects, fruits and vegetables—not supplements—were the key sources of these nutrients. In fact, clinical studies with supplements have proven how difficult it is to distinguish between the effect of a food and the effect of one of its many specific components. At best, such studies have produced disappointing results, and a few have even raised the possibility that high doses of a single antioxidant may be harmful. For example, the Physicians' Health Study found that beta-carotene supplements provided no protection against cancer, and two other studies found that beta-carotene supplements increase the incidence of lung cancer in smokers. In none of the three studies did beta-carotene supplements protect against CHD.

Some researchers hypothesize that the large amounts of beta-carotene in the supplements increased lung cancer incidence in these studies because the beta-carotene blocked the absorption of other carotenoids that are protective. This possibility underscores the potential dangers of overloading with one particular nutrient by taking large doses of supplements. Such studies should not stop people from eating foods that supply beta-carotene, which is only one of hundreds of carotenoids in foods. It is virtually impossible to get too much of any particular nutrient from foods alone.

Other carotenoids are also emerging as possibly protective against cancer and other disorders. For example, studies have suggested that tomatoes and tomato-based products (such as tomato sauce, tomato juice, and ketchup) are linked to a reduced risk of cancer, particularly prostate cancer. Tomatoes are a leading source of lycopene, the carotenoid that gives tomatoes their red color. In a recent study of the lycopene–cancer connection, researchers examined data from 47,365 men in the Health Professionals Follow-Up Study. The participants completed questionnaires about their diet, including their intake of tomato products such as tomato sauce as well as other dietary sources of lycopene (including such foods as watermelon and pink grapefruit). Over a 12-year period, men who ate at least two servings of tomato sauce per week had a 23% lower risk of prostate cancer than men who ate less than one serving per month. Eating two or more servings per week also reduced the risk of metastatic prostate cancer by 35%. Similarly, men with the highest lycopene intake had a 16% lower risk of prostate cancer than men with the lowest lycopene intake.

More studies are needed to firmly establish whether lycopene, alone or in combination with other dietary components, actually reduces prostate cancer risk. In the meantime, it is reasonable for men to consume tomato-based products and other foods with lycopene on a regular basis. The greatest protective effect of tomatoes appears to come from cooked tomato products, such as sauce, since cooking concentrates the lycopene content and increases its absorption. Watermelon is another good source of lycopene.

Selenium is a mineral that has been associated with a reduced risk of developing various cancers. Selenium acts indirectly as an antioxidant; it is an essential component of certain enzymes that inactivate free radicals. Research indicates that people with a high intake of this mineral, and those who live in areas where the selenium content of the soil is high, have a lower risk of lung, colon, and other cancers. Selenium is found in Brazil nuts, sunflower seeds, fish, turkey, wheat germ and other grains, fruits, and vegetables. The amount of selenium in plant foods depends on the amount of the mineral in the soil where the food is grown. Preliminary studies suggest that selenium supplements may help reduce cancer incidence, but further research is necessary.

Antioxidants and Other Disorders

A diet rich in carotenoids, especially lutein and zeaxanthin, has been linked to a reduced risk of developing macular degeneration, an age-related visual disorder that reduces central vision. The retina (the light-sensitive portion of the eye that receives and transmits visual impulses to the brain via the optic nerve) is rich in lutein and zeaxanthin, and studies suggest that these carotenoids protect the macula—the most sensitive portion of the retina—from damaging ultraviolet rays.

In October 2001, researchers from the Age-Related Eye Disease Study (AREDS) reported in the *Archives of Ophthalmology* that taking a combination of antioxidant vitamins and zinc reduced the rate of

NEW RESEARCH

Vitamin A Linked to Fractures

Older men with high amounts of vitamin A in their blood have an elevated risk of fractures, a new study indicates.

Swedish researchers analyzed blood levels of vitamin A in 2,322 men, age 49 to 51, in the early 1970s. After a follow-up of 30 years, men with high levels of vitamin A had a 1.6-fold increased risk of having a fracture anywhere in the body (including a 2.5-fold increased risk of hip fracture) compared with men who had average levels. Those with the highest vitamin A levels (e.g., men in the top 1%) had a sevenfold increased fracture risk compared with men who had average levels.

Cell and animal studies suggest that high doses of vitamin A inhibit the formation of bone and stimulate bone resorption. The current study indicates that a similar process may occur in humans and increase bone fragility.

Vitamin A supplementation and fortification of food with vitamin A "may be harmful in Western countries, where the life expectancy is high and the prevalence of osteoporosis is increasing," the author of an accompanying editorial writes.

Liver, fish, dairy products, fortified foods, and supplements are the main sources of vitamin A. To be safe, people should not consume more than the recommended dietary allowance of vitamin A—1,000 micrograms (mcg) for men and 800 mcg for women.

THE NEW ENGLAND JOURNAL OF MEDICINE
Volume 348, pages 287 and 347
January 23, 2003

Food Allergies: Sorting Through the Confusion

What appears to be a food allergy often isn't. Here's how to tell if you actually have one, and what to do about it.

One out of three people say that they have a food allergy or that they modify the family diet because a family member is thought to have a food allergy. In reality, however, only about 1% of adults in the United States suffers from a clinically proven food allergy.

The confusion surrounding food allergies may be due in part to the similarity between symptoms caused by a true food allergy and symptoms caused by food intolerance.

What Is a Food Allergy?

A food allergy is an abnormal response to a food that is triggered by the immune system. Symptoms of a food allergy can include the following: a tingling sensation in the mouth, swelling of the tongue and throat, rash, hives, eczema, abdominal cramps, vomiting, diarrhea, wheezing, difficulty breathing, and anaphylaxis (a severe allergic reaction that can be fatal if not treated quickly). Symptoms of a food allergy generally occur within a few minutes to an hour or two. Most people don't suffer extreme reactions; their allergic reactions to food are usually a temporary, albeit unpleasant, discomfort.

How the Allergic Reaction Occurs

An allergic reaction to a food happens when the immune system mistakenly believes that a food is harmful and attempts to protect the body. This reaction involves a specific sequence of events, beginning with the first ingestion of the allergen-containing food that stimulates the production and release of a type of protein called immunoglobulin E (IgE), an antibody that circulates through the bloodstream and binds to the surface of mast cells. The next time this same food is ingested, the IgE triggers the mast cells to produce massive amounts of chemicals such as histamine. The release of these chemicals, depending upon the location of the mast cells, will cause the person to experience various symptoms of food allergy. For example, if the targeted tissue is the ears, nose, and throat, the result may be difficulty breathing or swallowing; on the skin, the result can be hives; or in the gastrointestinal tract, the reaction may cause diarrhea.

The development of IgE in response to certain foods is an inherited predisposition. Studies show that people with food allergies often come from families in which allergies are common—not necessarily food allergies, perhaps other allergic reactions like asthma or hay fever.

Foods Commonly Linked to Food Allergies

While any food can cause an allergic reaction, eight common offenders are responsible for up to 90% of all food allergies. In children, milk, soy, eggs, wheat, peanuts, nuts, fish, and shellfish most commonly cause food allergies, while adults are more likely to be allergic to peanuts, nuts, and shellfish. Severe episodes that result in anaphylaxis are usually due to peanut or nut allergies. And while children can sometimes outgrow food allergies, adults usually do not.

How To Tell If You Have a Food Allergy

It is important to see your doctor if you note a pattern of symptoms after eating a certain food. Ideally, you should see your doctor during the allergic reaction, although this isn't always possible. Your doctor will ask for a detailed history of your symptoms and ask if you have a family history of food allergies. You also may be asked to keep a food diary to create a clear picture of your eating patterns.

After ruling out other medical causes of your symptoms, your doctor may conduct skin tests to determine your reaction to particular allergens, or he or she may administer a blood test to measure the presence of food-specific IgE in the blood. Keep in mind, however, that neither of these tests is 100% accurate.

Your doctor may also ask you to try an elimination diet. Food elimination involves the complete exclusion of the suspected food or foods from the diet for a week or two. If the symptoms go away when the food is eliminated and come back when the food is reintroduced, the doctor may make a diagnosis. However, this ap-

progression of age-related macular degeneration (AMD) in some people. The AREDS researchers studied 3,640 people, age 55 to 80, who had no AMD, early AMD in one or both eyes, intermediate AMD in one or both eyes, or advanced AMD in one eye. Neither antioxidants nor zinc, alone or in combination, reduced the risk of developing AMD in people without the disease or slowed its progres-

proach is not 100% foolproof either, particularly if a person is allergic to more than one food. This elimination technique cannot be used if the reactions are infrequent or severe.

The Best Treatments for Food Allergies

There are several approaches to treating food allergies, beginning with some relatively easy lifestyle changes such as avoidance and awareness.

Avoidance. Once you discover which food is causing symptoms, strict avoidance of the allergy-causing food is the best way to avoid a reaction. If someone has a life-threatening reaction to a certain food, the doctor will also advise the patient to avoid similar foods that might trigger this reaction. For example, in someone with an allergy to shrimp, tests will usually show that the person has a "cross-reactive" allergy to crab, lobster, and crayfish.

Awareness. It's important to know what's in the foods you buy. This can sometimes be tricky, because many allergy-producing foods such as peanuts, eggs, and milk, are present in foods one normally would not associate them with. Fortunately, food labels are required to list all ingredients (except spices, flavors, certain colors, and incidental additives). The Food Allergy and Anaphylaxis Network (FAAN) is a nonprofit organization that works to increase public awareness about food allergies. FAAN is encouraging food manufacturers to use simple, consumer-friendly terms on food labels. For example, the word "milk" or "egg" is clearer than casein, whey, or albumin. If a food contains an allergen that is not listed on the food label, the FDA will issue an immediate recall for that product.

When eating out, ask if any allergy-producing foods are used in the dishes you plan to order.

Medications. People who experience severe anaphylactic reactions may need to carry a prescription medication such as self-injectable adrenaline (epinephrine). They should also wear a medical alert bracelet or necklace stating that they have a food allergy.

Several medications are available to relieve food allergy symptoms that do not cause an anaphylactic reaction. Antihistamines can relieve gastrointestinal symptoms, hives, sneezing, or a runny nose; bronchodilators can relieve asthma symptoms. To date, no medication can be taken before eating a certain food to reliably prevent an allergic reaction to that food.

Consult your doctor to keep apprised of any new developments in the field of food allergy research to see what other options are available. For more information, contact the American Academy of Allergy, Asthma, and Immunology at www.aaaai.org or 800-822-2762; The Food Allergy and Anaphylaxis Network at www.foodallergy.org or 800-929-4040; or the Asthma and Allergy Foundation of America at www.aafa.org or 800-7-ASTHMA.

Common Types of Food Intolerance

A food intolerance is an adverse reaction to a food that does not involve an immune system response—a key factor in a clinically proven food allergy. Although it may be unpleasant, food intolerance is rarely dangerous. Food intolerance and its symptoms can have a variety of causes:

- Histamines, which are present naturally in certain foods such as wine, cheese, and some fish (particularly tuna and mackerel), can initiate a reaction that strongly resembles a true food allergy.
- Lactose intolerance, frequently confused with a food allergy, is a common disorder caused by an inability to digest the lactose present in most milk products. Symptoms of lactose intolerance (bloating, abdominal pain, and sometimes diarrhea) mimic those associated with a true food allergy.
- Food additives, flavor enhancers, and other substances such as sulfites can cause adverse allergy-like reactions.
- Ulcers and cancers of the gastrointestinal tract can produce symptoms similar to those of food allergies.

Many people with lactose intolerance are able to buy lactose-reduced dairy products or take tablets that contain lactase, the enzyme that helps the body digest lactose. Aside from this, there are no treatments for food intolerance besides avoiding the offending foods.

sion in those with early AMD. However, people with intermediate AMD or advanced AMD in one eye who took both antioxidants and zinc reduced their risk of progression to more advanced AMD by about 25%; in addition, these individuals lowered their risk of vision loss from AMD by 19%.

Because the supplements that were used in the AREDS study

contain larger dosages of vitamins and minerals than those present in a normal diet or a typical vitamin tablet, you should check with your primary care physician before starting to take any supplements. This caution applies especially to people receiving treatment for diabetes, heart disease, or cancer. In addition, the AREDS supplements may interfere with over-the-counter or prescription medications or interact with other dietary supplements or herbal preparations.

Finally, vitamin E may help to improve the immune system and memory in older people. One study found that extremely high doses of vitamin E—2,000 IU per day—slowed the progression of Alzheimer's disease (although no improvement in symptoms was noted in the patients). These possible effects are promising, but more research is needed. Make sure to check with your doctor before taking extra vitamin E if you are taking daily blood-thinning medications such as warfarin (Coumadin) or aspirin, because vitamin E, too, reduces the ability of the blood to clot.

Recommendations for Antioxidant Intake

1. Get most of your antioxidants from fruits and vegetables, not supplements. A diet containing five to nine servings of fruits and vegetables per day can easily provide an adequate amount of vitamin C, beta-carotene, other carotenoids, dietary fiber, and phytochemicals, as well as other vitamins and minerals. It's possible that the beneficial effect of antioxidants only occurs when they are consumed in combination with each other or with other substances, known and not known, in plant foods. Furthermore, the long-term effects of high-dose antioxidants are unknown and may include increased lung cancer risk in smokers; high-dose zinc can interfere with some medications and may produce gastrointestinal side effects.

2. Focus on dark green vegetables and orange, red, and yellow fruits and vegetables. Fruits and vegetables of these colors are the most nutritious. They provide substantial amounts of antioxidants and vitamin C, as well as other beneficial nutrients.

3. Be sure to get the RDA for vitamin C: 75 mg for women and 90 mg for men. These amounts are easily obtained through diet. The vitamin chart on pages 20–21 lists some common dietary sources.

4. Don't take selenium supplements. The difference between an adequate and a toxic dose of selenium is quite small. People concerned that they are not getting enough selenium might consider a multivitamin-mineral supplement that contains no more than the RDA for selenium (55 mcg).

PHYTOCHEMICALS

Fruits, vegetables, and other plant foods may protect against disease. From anthocyanins (the red pigment in strawberries and cherries) to allylic sulfides (which are responsible for the pungent flavor of garlic and onions), plant foods contain a plethora of chemical compounds that give them color and flavor and even protect them from insects. These compounds, termed phytochemicals, may be responsible for part of the disease-preventing effect of fruits and vegetables.

Phytochemicals have no traditional nutritive value—that is, they are not vitamins or minerals—but they may have positive effects on the body over the long term. These effects include inhibiting tumor formation, producing an anticoagulant effect, blocking the cancer-promoting effect of certain hormones, and lowering cholesterol levels.

As noted in the antioxidant section (see page 34), studies exploring the effects of supplements (other than possibly vitamin E) have failed to show that a high intake of isolated nutrients reduces the risk of disease. These observations leave open the possibility that other substances in plant foods, namely phytochemicals, may be important in disease prevention, either on their own or in combination with the antioxidants.

Phytochemicals are found in a wide variety of plant foods, and indeed many different phytochemicals are often present in a single food—for example, more than 170 have been identified in oranges. The vast number of compounds in fruits, vegetables, grains, and legumes makes it nearly impossible for supplements to substitute for a healthy diet. While the beneficial effects, if any, of phytochemicals have yet to be proven, the following show some promise for disease prevention.

Allylic sulfides. Found in onions and garlic, these substances may enhance immune function, help the body to excrete cancer-causing compounds, and interfere with the development of tumors.

Flavonoids. These compounds function as antioxidants. They may be involved in several actions, including extending the life of vitamin C, inhibiting tumor development, preventing the oxidation of LDL cholesterol, and controlling inflammation. Various flavonoids are found in a host of fruits and vegetables, as well as in red wine, red and purple grape juice, and green and black tea.

Indoles, isothiocyanates, and sulforaphane. In 1992, researchers at Johns Hopkins found that broccoli, kale, brussels sprouts, and

NEW RESEARCH

Fruits and Vegetables Better for Health Than Supplements

Many people take dietary supplements in an effort to reduce their risk of cancer, heart disease, and other health problems. However, a recent review article proposes that the additive effects of the chemicals present in whole foods offers more health benefits than supplements of the individual compounds.

Researchers mention several examples showing that fruits and vegetables offer superior health benefits over dietary supplements. For example, 128 of 156 studies found that people who ate a diet rich in fruits and vegetables had half the risk of most types of cancer as people who ate a diet low in fruits and vegetables. By contrast, supplements of the single phytochemical beta-carotene (present in green and yellow fruits and vegetables) did not protect against cancer in several studies.

The researchers conclude that the phytochemicals and other bioactive substances contained in fruits and vegetables have additive effects, working together to protect against cancer and other diseases. They also write that "pills or tablets simply cannot mimic this balanced natural combination of phytochemicals present in fruit and vegetables."

AMERICAN JOURNAL OF CLINICAL NUTRITION
Volume 78, page 517S
September 2003

other members of the cabbage family (also known as cruciferous vegetables) contain a potent substance—sulforaphane—that stimulates cells to produce cancer-fighting enzymes. Since then, indoles and isothiocyanates, also present in cruciferous vegetables, have been found to act in a similar manner.

Phenolic acids. Ellagic acid, ferulic acid, and other phenolic acids may prevent damage to DNA. They are found in strawberries, raspberries, tomatoes, citrus fruits, whole grains, and nuts.

Phytoestrogens. Phytoestrogens are plant substances that are converted to estrogen-like compounds by bacteria in the intestine. They are present in many common foods, especially soybeans and soy products such as tofu and soy milk. Lignans and isoflavones are examples of phytoestrogens. Researchers believe that these compounds may help prevent breast cancer by stopping the estrogen produced in the body from entering cells. In addition, the estrogen-like effect produced by these compounds may temper the production of testosterone in men and thus help to thwart prostate cancer. Some reports also suggest that women who eat a lot of soy products have fewer hot flashes associated with menopause.

Soy products may also lower blood cholesterol levels. In a meta-analysis of 38 studies where soy protein replaced animal protein in people's diets, eating an average of 47 g of soy protein per day lowered levels of total cholesterol by about 9%, LDL cholesterol by 13%, and triglycerides by 11%. It is not known whether soy products lower cholesterol levels simply by replacing saturated fats with unsaturated fats (soybeans derive 38% of their calories from fat, mostly unsaturated) or from the isoflavones in soybeans.

Saponins. These sugar-like compounds have an antibacterial effect. Saponins may strengthen the immune system, prevent microbial and fungal infections, and fight viruses. They are found in potatoes, tomatoes, legumes, oats, and spinach.

Recommendations for Phytochemical Intake

1. Follow a plant-based diet. Eat five to nine servings of fruits and vegetables and at least six servings of grain products each day, and consume legumes several times a week. Vary the choices to get a wide range of phytochemicals, but focus on dark green vegetables, red and orange fruits and vegetables, and whole grains.

2. Season foods with herbs and spices. Such seasonings also contain phytochemicals. Try using garlic, shallots, ginger, basil, oregano, parsley, rosemary, cumin, curry powder, cayenne pepper, red chili pepper, and cinnamon, to name a few.

NEW RESEARCH

People Who Eat Meatless Diets May Live Longer

Eating little or no meat may increase your life span, according to a recent review article. Other studies have shown that life expectancy is up to two years longer in countries that have a lower meat intake than in the United States, where only about 6% of people eat a meatless diet.

Researchers analyzed six studies of meatless or low-meat diets and life span. Four studies found that people who ate little or no meat were 12% to 56% less likely to die during the follow-up (from 5 to 26 years) than people who ate meat at least once a week. One study found a nonsignificant decrease in the risk of death for vegetarians; a sixth study found no link. In two of the studies that showed a link, people who followed a low-meat or meatless diet for at least 20 years lived an extra 3.6 years.

The researchers note that some people who follow a vegetarian diet may also have other healthy habits—like exercising and not smoking—that increase life span. But they point out that most of the six studies adjusted the results for some, but not all, of these factors. Although vegetarians avoid the unhealthy components of meat (such as saturated fat), they could benefit from a high intake of healthy meat alternatives, like legumes, vegetables, nuts, and soy foods, the researchers suggest.

AMERICAN JOURNAL OF CLINICAL NUTRITION
Volume 78, page 526S
September 2003

3. Incorporate soy products. Tofu, soy protein, soymilk, soy flour, soy butter, and edamame (edible green soybeans) are all examples. The amounts of soy protein vary: 8 oz. of soymilk has 4 to 10 g; 4 oz. of tofu has 8 to 13 g; 1 oz. of soy flour has 10 to 13 g; ½ cup of textured soy protein (TVP or TSP) has 11 g. Many soy products taste better than they did several years ago; "veggie" burgers, for example, have become popular, though not all vegetarian burgers are made from tofu (check the label). Tofu and other soy products are mild tasting and pick up the flavor of the foods they are cooked with; try mixing TVP into meat loaf, casserole, or chili recipes. Soy flour can substitute for up to one quarter of the total flour in baking recipes. Tofu can be stir-fried with vegetables or added to soups, and soy butter can be spread on bread in place of peanut butter.

ENHANCED FOODS

As part of an effort to ensure that people eat well, and to help with disease prevention, several areas of food research are devoted to improving the types of foods we eat. These foods include ones that have been enriched or fortified with the addition of healthy components, as well as foods that have been genetically modified to provide certain nutrients. The concept of using food as a way to prevent disease is not new. Beginning in the 1920s, iodine was added to salt to prevent goiters; later, milk was fortified with vitamin D to prevent rickets.

Enriched food. An enriched food contains nutrients that are added to increase the amount originally present or to replace nutrients lost during processing. An example is white rice that is enriched with B vitamins and iron that were lost during processing.

Fortified food. Foods that have been "fortified" have had vitamins and/or minerals added to them; they are marketed to promote health and prevent disease. The added nutrients were not present in the original food or were present in lower amounts. Such foods include folic acid-fortified wheat products, orange juice fortified with calcium, and vitamin D-fortified milk.

Functional food. Although the U.S. Food and Drug Administration (FDA) has made no legal definition of functional foods (see www.cfsan.fda.gov/label.html), many groups use this term to refer to foods with specific health benefits that go beyond traditional nutritional effects. Because there is no uniform definition, the term can be applied in different ways. It is sometimes used to refer only

How To Avoid a Foodborne Illness

Foodborne illnesses are estimated to cause 76 million infections, 300,000 hospitalizations, and 5,000 or more deaths annually—but there are many ways to prevent them.

The most common forms of foodborne illness are infections caused by microscopic agents that thrive in or on food that has not been properly handled. Unwashed, raw, or undercooked foods are the most vulnerable to this type of contamination. In this country, the usual contaminants are bacteria (including various species of Shigella, Salmonella, and Staphylococcus; *Campylobacter jejuni*, *Bacillus cereus,* and certain strains of *Escherichia coli*) and viruses (most commonly the Norwalk or Norwalk-like viruses).

Although many people assume that all foodborne illnesses are "food poisoning," food poisoning is only one type of foodborne illness. True food poisoning is caused by a harmful contaminant, such as a toxin or a chemical. For example, food poisoning can result from deadly toxins produced by poisonous mushrooms or by the bacterium *Clostridium botulinum* (which results in botulism).

Food-related infections can also be caused by parasites, but such infections are more likely to be encountered abroad in areas where food-handling practices are less stringent than in the United States.

Preventing Illness at Home

Proper food-handling practices and personal hygiene are key to preventing foodborne illness. Here are some prevention tips you should follow when choosing, storing, preparing, and serving food.

Shopping

- Avoid packaging that is ripped or leaky when buying perishable products.
- Select perishable items last.
- Choose items that have not reached their expiration date.
- Pass up cans that are bulging or dented.
- Do not purchase fresh, prestuffed, whole poultry.
- Drink only pasteurized milk and juice.
- Check fresh food for mold.

Storage

- Refrigerate food at 40° F or below; freeze food at 0° F or below (use a freezer thermometer).
- Refrigerate oils containing garlic or herbs.
- Store raw meat, poultry, and seafood away from other foods to prevent bacteria from spreading; seal these foods in containers or bags to prevent raw juices from dripping onto other foods.
- Freeze or cook fresh poultry, seafood, and ground meat within two days of purchase. Freeze or cook whole cuts of meat within three to five days.
- Avoid overstuffing the refrigerator, so that air may circulate around food.
- Save cooked leftovers for no more than four days.

Preparation

- Wash hands thoroughly with soap and water for 20 seconds before and after handling food.
- Thaw frozen foods in the refrigerator (never at room temperature), then cook immediately. For faster thawing, use the microwave or submerge foods in cold water in a sealed container; cook immediately afterwards.
- Always refrigerate food that is being marinated.
- Avoid cross-contamination: Use one cutting board and set of utensils to prepare any raw meat, fish, poultry, or eggs for a meal. Use a separate cutting board and utensils for all other ingredients (such as vegetables or bread).
- Use strict sanitary procedures when home canning. Boil home-canned food before eating, if possible, to destroy any potential microbes.
- Clean fruits and vegetables thoroughly with water before eating.
- Sanitize cutting boards and countertops with a solution of 1 teaspoon of chlorine bleach in 1 quart of water.

to enhanced foods, such as enriched and fortified foods, and sometimes the term refers to natural foods with probable benefits. An example is the tomato as a source of lycopene.

Nutraceuticals. Pharmaceutical companies have also started to manufacture functional foods that are intended to have drug-like effects. Broadly known as nutraceuticals, these functional foods rack up billions of dollars in sales. Fruit juice and iced tea with

If You Suspect Foodborne Illness
Recognizing symptoms of foodborne illness and knowing when to see a doctor or administer self-care can minimize risk and ensure a safe recovery.

The symptoms of food-related infections are similar, regardless of the underlying pathogen. They typically include some combination of nausea, vomiting, and diarrhea, sometimes with fever. Symptoms generally develop within 12 to 72 hours of eating tainted food. Most cases are mild and resolve spontaneously. However, severe infections can cause high fever and significant dehydration.

Failing to recognize symptoms and to treat a food-related illness can have serious, even deadly consequences, particularly in vulnerable people, such as young children and the elderly. Other high-risk people include those with a compromised immune system (including people taking antirejection drugs after an organ transplant), a chronic medical problem such as coronary heart disease or diabetes, and people undergoing certain medical treatments such as long-term corticosteroid therapy, radiation therapy, or chemotherapy.

High-risk people should see a physician as soon as a food-related infection is suspected. Healthy people should see their physician if they have bloody diarrhea, weight loss, a fever of 101° F or higher, severe abdominal pain, neurological symptoms (including motor weakness, numbness, or tingling), or prolonged diarrhea. Treatment includes bed rest and fluids, along with oral antibiotics when appropriate. Very high-risk people and those with severe infections may require hospitalization.

Healthy people with mild to moderate symptoms can usually treat themselves with bed rest and fluids. Over-the-counter antidiarrheal medications, such as loperamide (Imodium A-D) and bismuth (Pepto-Bismol, Bismatrol), may relieve cramps and minimize diarrhea. However, loperamide may worsen the effects of some bacterial infections (including Salmonella, Shigella, and *Campylobacter jejuni*) and should not be used without consulting a doctor if a food-related infection is suspected. In any case, neither medication should be taken for more than 48 hours.

To help prevent a mass outbreak of foodborne illness, notify the local health department if the contaminated food was served at a large gathering, a restaurant, or other facility, or if the food was purchased at a commercial establishment.

Cooking

- Thoroughly cook meat, poultry, seafood, and eggs. (Cook eggs until the yolk is firm.) Use a meat thermometer to ensure proper internal cooking temperatures of meat, poultry, and casseroles; insert the thermometer into the thickest part of the food, as far as possible from bone, fat, or gristle.
- Do not serve raw or lightly cooked sprouts. Avoid them or cook them thoroughly.
- Reheat foods to an internal temperature of 165° F.
- Cook steaks, roasts, and chops of beef, veal, and lamb to an internal temperature of 145° F; all cuts of pork, to 160° F.
- Cook whole poultry, as well as poultry thighs and wings, to an internal temperature of 180° F; breasts, to 170° F.
- Cook ground meat to an internal temperature of 160° F; ground poultry, to 165° F.

Serving

- Hold hot foods at 140° F or higher and cold foods at 40° F or lower.
- Use warming trays and chafing dishes to serve hot foods at a buffet; hold cold foods on ice.
- Serve food on clean plates that have not touched raw meat, fish, poultry, or eggs.
- Refrigerate foods promptly after serving. Discard perishables left at room temperature for two hours or more; one hour if the room or outdoor temperature is 90° F or above.
- Never give honey to a baby because of the potential for botulism poisoning.

added herbs like ginkgo biloba are examples of nutraceuticals. Experts predict that nutraceuticals could be one of the biggest growth areas in food production. The incredible increase in the number of nutraceuticals on the market in the past few years does not indicate that their health claims have been substantiated. There is little evidence that these products are beneficial, and many of the ingredients used in nutraceuticals have not been tested in clinical trials.

Genetically modified food. Genetic modification of food is another food science initiative, in which new genes are introduced into crops to improve their health benefits or make them hardier. For example, research is under way to reprogram plant genes to reduce unhealthy fats, yield biodegradable plastics, or act as antigens (a kind of edible vaccine against infectious organisms).

However, genetic modification of food crops has been the subject of a great deal of controversy, and many countries in Europe have banned the import of such foods. Critics argue that the unpredictable consequences of genetic modifications may have a serious impact on the ecosystem. Although genetically altered foods have been tested and are considered safe, long-term studies have not examined the environmental impact.

ORGANIC FOODS

More Americans are turning to organic foods out of a concern for the environment as well as a desire to minimize their exposure to certain chemicals in their food. As a result, the market for organic foods is thriving. Over the past decade, consumer demand for organic foods has increased 20% or more each year in the United States. The Food Marketing Institute estimates that approximately 40% of all U.S. shoppers have purchased at least one organic product. A diverse array of organic goods—from produce to frozen foods—is readily available to consumers, and the popularity of organic foods is expected to continue.

A national definition of the term organic was recently established by the federal government. This definition encompasses a set of standards that governs the production, labeling, and marketing of organic foods. In order to be called organic, a food must be produced without the use of bioengineered foods, herbicides, irradiation, pesticides, synthetic fertilizers, or sewage sludge. Organic livestock must be raised on 100% organic feed, and antibiotics and growth hormones are prohibited. To find out if a food is organic, check the label for a "USDA Certified Organic" seal. (USDA stands for U.S. Department of Agriculture.)

While all organic foods carry the basic seal of approval, labels identifying foods as organic differ according to the quantity of organic ingredients the food contains:

- **100% organic** means the food contains only organically produced raw or processed ingredients, with the exception of water and salt.

- **Organic** indicates that 95% of the ingredients are organically produced and the remaining 5% are from the USDA-approved national list.
- **Made with organic ingredients** denotes that at least 70% of the ingredients in the product are organic. For more information on organic food labels and regulations, visit the USDA's National Organic Program Web site at www.ams.usda.gov/nop.

Currently, there is no scientific evidence that organic foods are safer, better in quality, or more nutritious than conventional foods. In addition, although many consumers perceive organic foods as healthier than conventional foods, a USDA Certified Organic seal does not signify freshness, enhanced taste, or superior quality or nutritional content. Nor does organic guarantee a food is pesticide free: Up to 5% pesticide residues are permitted in organic foods.

FOOD SAFETY

U.S. consumers have one of the safest supplies of food in the world, but the increasing global exchange of food has recently highlighted the risk of foodborne diseases and suggests the need for an international agreement on standards for food production. In any case, research continues on ways to prevent food contamination.

The National Animal and Disease Center is developing several faster and more advanced tests to identify foodborne pathogens, and the USDA and FDA are supporting a "farm-to-table" approach to eliminate and control foodborne toxins at all steps along the chain of food production and consumption. One recent advance uses antibodies that bind to toxins produced by bacteria and fungi (molds) to measure the content of the organisms in foods. Referred to as ELISA (enzyme-linked immunosorbent assay), these highly sensitive tests can identify trace amounts of a toxin and take less time than traditional disease-detection strategies. ELISA test kits to detect bacterial toxins in food are currently in development for use by farmers.

Other strategies to fight foodborne bacteria are evolving from developments in genetic therapy and molecular biology. For example, scientists found that inactivating a gene called DAM can disarm the ability of a strain of Salmonella to cause disease. These approaches to detection and prevention, combined with proper food preparation and refrigeration techniques, should help to further improve the safety of our food supply.

Weight Control

In addition to adopting good overall nutritional habits, one of the most important ways to preserve good health is to control your weight. Rates of overweight and obesity are higher than ever, according to the Centers for Disease Control and Prevention, which estimates that more than 6 in 10 American adults are overweight or obese. By shedding pounds, overweight people can reduce their risk of type 2 diabetes, high blood pressure, and coronary heart disease (CHD). Losing weight may lower levels of low density lipoprotein (LDL) cholesterol, which is often referred to as "bad" cholesterol. Losing weight can also lower levels of triglycerides and even increase high density lipoprotein (HDL) cholesterol, referred to as "good" cholesterol. In addition, weight loss can help reduce the risk of osteoarthritis and gallstones.

In theory, weight control is a simple matter of balancing energy intake (the calories supplied by food) with energy output (the calories expended by physical activity and metabolism). To lose weight, you need to expend more energy than you take in. In practice, however, the task is clearly not that simple. Obesity—the medical term for excessive amounts of body fat—is a chronic condition, like hypertension or diabetes. While the basic principle of energy balance remains true, several mechanisms—genetic, metabolic, and environmental—control how much you eat and how your body uses and stores energy.

Even if some of the components involved in weight regulation are beyond your control, environmental factors have a significant impact. By manipulating these factors to your advantage, you can successfully lose weight and keep it off.

METABOLISM

A certain amount of calories are needed to supply the energy required for metabolism and everyday activities. When more calories are consumed than are needed, these extra calories are stored primarily as fat—whether the calories come from fat, carbohydrates, or proteins, though dietary fat is converted into body fat most efficiently.

During digestion, enzymes in the small intestine break down carbohydrates into simple sugars like glucose, proteins into amino acids, and triglycerides (dietary fat) into fatty acids and glycerol. Simple sugars and amino acids are rapidly absorbed from the small intestine into the bloodstream. The liver converts other sugars, like fructose and lactose, into glucose, which is used as a source of energy. Amino acids can be used as an energy source but serve mainly as building blocks for body proteins. Fatty acids combine with bile salts to form tiny droplets that promote their entry into cells in the intestinal wall, where they are again formed into triglycerides. The triglycerides are packaged into transport lipoproteins called chylomicrons, which carry the triglycerides to the adipose tissue (fat) for storage of any triglycerides not immediately used to provide energy.

Any excess carbohydrates and protein not immediately used for energy are converted to glycogen and triglycerides in the liver. These triglycerides are transported from the liver on another lipoprotein (very low density lipoprotein) for storage in various parts of the body in individual adipose tissue cells, located just beneath the skin or around the intestines.

To store more fat, the body either creates more fat cells (a process called hyperplasia, which generally occurs only in childhood-onset obesity, during pregnancy, or with rapid weight gain in adults) or enlarges existing fat cells (hypertrophy, the primary way that adults increase their adipose tissue). If faced with a shortage of calories—as when a person diets—the body uses the fat stored in these cells as a source of energy. Unfortunately, once fat cells are formed they can shrink, but they are not eliminated.

FACTORS THAT AFFECT BODY WEIGHT

Controllable factors—such as a high-calorie diet, inappropriate psychological responses to food, and a lack of exercise—play a critical role in the development of obesity. But research has confirmed that more is involved than just a lack of willpower or a sedentary lifestyle.

Risk Factors That Cannot Be Changed

Although these factors are beyond your control, their impact on weight can be modified by changes in diet and physical activity.

Heredity. Studies show that 80% of children born to two obese parents will themselves become obese, compared with 14% of children born to normal-weight parents. Research on identical twins shows similarly high rates of inheritance. However, studies comparing the weights of adoptees with the weights of their biological and adopted parents indicate that genetic factors are responsible for only about one third of the variance in weight, a figure experts believe is more accurate. Heredity seems to influence the number of fat cells in the body, how much and where fat is stored, and the resting

NEW RESEARCH

Obesity Shortens Life Expectancy

Obesity has a profound impact on life span, especially among younger adults. Data also suggest that the life-threatening effects of being excessively overweight are most pronounced in white men.

Investigators reached these conclusions after they analyzed national health databases and estimated the relationship between obesity and years of life lost based on several variables, including body mass index (BMI).

The life expectancy of severely obese (BMI greater than 45) white men at age 20 to 30 was an average of 13 years shorter than that of their normal-weight counterparts. This represents a 22% reduction in expected remaining life. Severely obese white women in the same age range lost an average of eight years of life. Obesity didn't begin to affect life span for any age group until BMI reached 32 in black men and 37 in black women.

The authors of an accompanying editorial praised the study for underscoring the dangers of obesity. But they cautioned that the assertion that blacks are less susceptible to the negative effects of excess weight are probably inaccurate—the result of limitations in statistical analysis—and that blacks should not assume that being overweight does them no harm.

JOURNAL OF THE AMERICAN MEDICAL ASSOCIATION
Volume 289, page 187
January 8, 2003

Weight and Longevity

Being overweight or obese can reduce your life expectancy, but even modest weight loss may help you live longer.

Obesity—which is linked to high blood pressure, diabetes, coronary heart disease, stroke, and cancer—is believed to cause more than 280,000 deaths annually in the United States. If current trends continue, obesity will soon overtake smoking as the number one preventable cause of death.

New research shows that obesity in middle-aged adults cuts life span dramatically. A 2003 analysis of the Framingham Heart Study suggests that middle-aged adults who are overweight or obese have shorter life expectancies than normal-weight adults. Published in the *Annals of Internal Medicine,* the 3,500-person study found that 40-year-old men and women, who were obese but did not smoke, were likely to die six to seven years earlier on average than their normal-weight counterparts. Obese smokers were likely to die 13½ years sooner than normal-weight nonsmokers.

Another 2003 study by researchers at Johns Hopkins, which analyzed data from a previous study, found that obesity in young adults is associated with the greatest reduction in life expectancy.

Even Modest Weight Loss Helps

But here's the good news: In recent years, research has found that losing as little as 10% of body weight, or sometimes even less, can improve your health. Small weight losses decrease the risk of a wide range of obesity-related illnesses ranging from coronary heart disease and diabetes to some kinds of cancer. The health payoffs from a modest weight loss may be due to the reduction in abdominal fat, which increases the risk of cardiovascular disease.

Extreme Calorie Restriction Is Not a Good Idea

Although studies have shown that animals placed on severe calorie-restricted diets throughout adulthood live 30% to 40% longer than animals kept on regular diets, it is not yet known if humans can reap similar benefits. Furthermore, calorie restrictions as drastic as those used in animal research (often 40% or more of normal calorie intake) are not practical on a long-term basis for people—and could be dangerous, particularly for the frail elderly and many people with chronic illnesses. And human studies on severe energy-restricted diets, such as very low (less than 800) calorie diets, show that the significant weight losses in the short term are followed by poor long-term maintenance of those losses.

Slow and Steady Is Best

Selecting an attainable, modest goal is a sensible start to a weight-loss program and can provide positive reinforcement when you succeed. In general, a gradual weight loss of 1 to 2 pounds per week is considered safe. To achieve this goal, you will need to begin by reducing your calorie intake. In general, decreasing calorie consumption by 250 to 500 calories daily, especially in conjunction with a modest increase in exercise, will result in weight loss of 1 to 2 pounds a week.

The important thing in achieving your weight loss goal is to be patient. Keep in mind, for example, that if you lose 3 pounds and your goal is 10, you are 30% toward your goal. When you add exercise to your weight-loss program, the calorie reduction can be less. The following chart illustrates the time it would take to attain a loss of 10% of body weight, at a rate of 1½ pounds per week. Be sure to consult your physician before embarking on any weight loss plan.

Current Weight	Goal Weight (10% reduction)	Weeks to Goal
140	126	9
150	135	10
160	144	11
170	153	11
180	162	12
190	171	13
200	180	13
210	189	14
220	198	15
230	207	15

metabolic rate. About 80% of obese children become obese adults, though only 20% of obese adults were obese as children.

A number of genes appear to be responsible for the regulation of body weight. A major advance occurred in 1994 when researchers at Rockefeller University discovered that mutations in a gene—termed the obesity (ob) gene—in one strain of mice prevented them from producing leptin, a hormone normally manufactured by adipose tissue cells and released into the bloodstream to inform the brain about the body's level of fat stores. When this communication system works correctly, the hypothalamic area of the brain responds to leptin by reducing appetite and speeding up metabolism to maintain a normal level of body fat. Because mice with the mutated ob gene did not produce leptin, their brains continued to prompt the storage of fat and they became obese. When leptin was injected into these obese mice, they quickly lost weight through a combination of decreased food intake and increased activity.

Mice who had no mutation but had simply been overfed lost some weight with leptin injections, but they lost much less weight than the leptin-lacking mice. A second strain of obese mice (db) had high leptin levels but did not respond to leptin because of a mutation in the gene for the leptin receptor in the hypothalamus (the site in the brain that normally receives the leptin message). Unraveling the links between leptin and weight may lead to the development of more effective drugs for weight loss.

Metabolism. This is the process that extracts and utilizes energy (measured in calories) from food. Even at rest, energy is needed for many functions, such as respiration, heart contractions, and cell repair and growth. The amount of energy used for these basic functions while a person is awake and at rest is known as the resting metabolic rate (RMR), which accounts for about 70% of energy utilization each day (although this percentage is lower in physically active individuals). RMR is affected by weight, age, and the ratio of lean tissue (muscle) to adipose tissue (fat), since muscle is metabolically more active than fat—that is, muscle utilizes more energy even at rest. RMR is also in part genetically determined.

Food intake itself generates energy expenditure because energy is needed to digest food, absorb nutrients, and store excess calories as body fat. This process—called the thermic effect of food, or thermogenesis—accounts for 10% to 15% of the body's total daily energy expenditure. Some research suggests that obese people require slightly less energy for thermogenesis, and so more of the calories they eat are stored as body fat rather than used to process food.

Whether or not obese people have an abnormally slow metabolism is a matter of controversy. Because it takes more energy to maintain a greater body mass, a person who weighs 200 lbs. has a higher RMR than one who weighs 150 lbs. In addition, a heavier person expends more calories than a leaner one for any given physical activity. But even when people of the same height, weight, age, sex, and lean body mass are compared, RMR may vary by 20% or more. Consequently, someone who would be predicted to use 1,200 calories through RMR may actually use anywhere from 1,080 to 1,320 calories. This variability could explain why two people who weigh the same may require different amounts of calories to maintain, lose, or gain weight.

Set point theory. According to this theory, each person has a predetermined level of body fat. How the body controls its fat stores is unknown, but the regulatory mechanism, sometimes called the adipostat, is probably located in the hypothalamus. (Other regions of the brain may also play a role.) The adipostat monitors body fat stores, possibly through the actions of leptin on its hypothalamic receptor, and works to maintain the prescribed level of fat, or set point, by adjusting appetite, physical activity, and RMR to conserve or expend energy. Thus, actions perceived to be voluntary, such as eating and physical activity, may be subtly controlled by the set point mechanism.

Factors That Can Be Changed

The following known factors are amenable to individual control.

Dietary intake. Eating more calories than you expend is an important cause of obesity. In fact, regardless of genetic predisposition or any other factors, you cannot gain weight without consuming more calories than you burn. Even small excesses in calorie intake—too small to measure accurately in the most rigorous study—can contribute to obesity over the long term. For example, a person who overeats by just 25 calories a day will consume 9,125 excess calories over the course of a year and so will gain 2½ lbs. (a pound of body fat is equivalent to 3,500 calories). A woman weighing 125 lbs. who starts this pattern at age 20 would weigh 175 lbs. by the time she is 40.

To point to overeating as the cause of obesity is overly simplistic, however. It does not explain why one 125-lb. woman needs 1,800 calories a day to meet her body's energy needs and avoid losing weight, while another 125-lb. woman struggles to avoid gaining weight on 1,200 calories a day.

Numerous other factors contribute to weight gain, including RMR and physical activity. Nevertheless, obese people must be consuming more calories than required by their individual make-ups and activity levels; otherwise they would not store excess body fat. A reduction in calorie intake is essential for weight loss.

Physical activity. Variations in physical activity can have a tremendous impact on total daily energy expenditure. A sedentary person may burn just a few hundred calories above RMR while going about daily activities (performing household chores or walking to the mailbox, for example), whereas an athlete can burn an additional 3,000 calories each day through vigorous exercise. Regular exercise not only burns calories, but also builds lean muscle mass and raises RMR because muscle requires more energy for maintenance. A low level of activity may be the most important factor responsible for the high and rising rate of obesity in the United States.

Behavioral and psychological issues. Several psychological factors affect weight control. The message to eat often comes from external cues rather than hunger—noon means it's time for lunch, for example. Food and emotions are closely linked; many people use food for comfort or to release tension. Obese people often eat quickly, and eating too fast can lead to taking in more calories than are needed to satisfy hunger. The amount of exercise a person engages in is also shaped by habit and attitudes toward physical activity. Some studies suggest that lean people may expend more energy than obese people in ordinary activities, as well as during formal exercise. For example, lean people may walk around (rather than sit) while on the phone, or may take the stairs rather than an elevator or escalator.

Hormonal (endocrine) abnormalities. An underactive thyroid (hypothyroidism) is often a layperson's explanation for obesity, but even when present, hypothyroidism is rarely a primary cause. Other conditions that may affect weight include polycystic ovary disease; tumors of the pituitary or adrenal glands; an insufficient production of sex hormones; and insulin-producing tumors of the pancreas. Nevertheless, although they are uncommon, these disorders need to be ruled out by a thorough medical evaluation before determining the best course of action to achieve weight loss.

MEDICAL CONSEQUENCES OF OBESITY

Overweight and obesity are linked with an increased risk of life-threatening conditions, such as type 2 diabetes, stroke, CHD, and cancer. The complications of excessive weight and obesity are a leading cause of preventable deaths, second only to tobacco-related complications. Current research indicates that in the United States approximately 300,000 deaths a year may be attributed to obesity.

NEW RESEARCH

Obesity, Diabetes Rates Rise Again

Continuing a trend that began in the 1990s, the percentage of people in the United States who are obese or have diabetes rose in 2001, investigators from the Centers for Disease Control and Prevention report.

In 2001, nearly 21% of adults (equivalent to 44.3 million Americans) were obese (i.e., a body mass index [BMI] of 30 or greater), up from 20% in 2000 and 12% in 1991. Also, about 2% of the U.S. adult population was morbidly obese (a BMI of 40 or greater) in 2001. In addition, about 8% of American adults were diagnosed with diabetes in 2001, up from 7% in 2000 and 5% in 1991.

These results were based on telephone interviews with 195,005 Americans, age 18 and older. Because people often underestimate their weight and overestimate their height, the actual rates of obesity are probably much higher. A recent study that measured people's weight and height, rather than obtaining self-reports, found an obesity rate of 30%. The rate of diabetes is also likely an underestimate, since about 35% of diabetes cases are undiagnosed.

Obesity and diabetes are preventable health problems. Programs to "promote a balanced diet, increase physical activity, and maintain weight control must be national priorities," the researchers write.

JOURNAL OF THE AMERICAN MEDICAL ASSOCIATION
Volume 289, page 76
January 1, 2003

The Obesity-Cancer Connection

More than 90,000 cancer deaths a year could be prevented if American adults maintained a healthy weight.

An impressive amount of scientific evidence has established obesity—defined as a body mass index (BMI) of 30 or more—as a risk factor for developing various types of cancer. Obesity also increases the risk of dying of cancer, even for those forms of cancer for which obesity is not already an established risk factor. A 2003 study by the American Cancer Society provides new evidence for this connection: As many as one in five cancer deaths each year among adults age 50 and over in the United States can be directly attributed to excess body weight. The message for Americans? Thousands of cancer deaths could be prevented if people lost weight.

Obesity and Cancer Risk

Obesity is a known risk factor for cancers of the breast, colon and rectum, endometrium (lining of the uterus), esophagus, and kidney.

Breast Cancer. The most common cancer in women, breast cancer is linked to obesity in postmenopausal women. Researchers estimate that obese women have a 50% greater chance than nonobese women of developing breast cancer after the menopause.

Colon and Rectal Cancer. The third leading cancer in men and women, colon and rectal cancer has been associated with several unhealthy aspects of the Western diet. However, obesity is the only recognized diet-related risk factor. Studies suggest that obesity doubles the risk of colorectal cancer in men and in premenopausal women.

Endometrial Cancer. The fourth most common cancer in women, endometrial cancer is linked to obesity in both premenopausal and postmenopausal women. Researchers estimate that obese women are three times more likely to develop endometrial cancer than women who are not obese.

Esophageal Cancer. Obesity is a known risk factor for developing a particular form of esophageal cancer, called adenocarcinoma, which arises from chronic damage to the lower esophagus.

Kidney Cancer. Although little information is available regarding the relationship between diet and kidney cancer, obesity has been identified as a risk factor. Obesity is thought to play a role in the development of one third of all kidney cancers in the United States.

The Risk of Dying of Cancer

The recent American Cancer Society study found that a large percentage of cancer deaths can be directly attributed to excess body weight.

At the start of this study, BMI was assessed in over 900,000 cancer-free American adults. Over a 16-year follow-up period, deaths from cancer were noted and then correlated to BMI. After accounting for other factors related to cancer deaths, such as age and physical activity, the investigators discovered a powerful relationship between cancer deaths and excess body weight: Participants who were overweight or obese were more likely than their normal-weight counterparts to die of any one of a large variety of cancers—non-Hodgkin's lymphoma, multiple myeloma, and cancer of the breast, cervix, colon and rectum, esophagus, gallbladder, kidney, liver, ovary, pancreas, prostate, stomach, or uterus.

Furthermore, the investigators found that the risk of dying increased as BMI increased. For example, women classified as overweight (a BMI of 25 to 29) at the beginning of the study were 50% more likely to die of uterine cancer than women of normal weight (a BMI under 25). Even worse, the risk of dying of uterine cancer more than doubled for obese women with a BMI of 30 to 39; and the risk was more than six times higher among morbidly obese women with a BMI of 40 or higher. In fact, both the heaviest men and women in the study had the highest risk: Men and women with a BMI of 40 or greater were 52% and 62%, respectively, more likely to die of cancer than normal-weight participants.

Altogether, the investigators estimate that excess body weight in the United States may contribute to 14% of all cancer deaths in men age 50 and over and to 20% of all cancer deaths in women age 50 and over. The compelling findings from this study suggest that if American adults maintained a healthy weight (a BMI

Studies show that mortality rates are substantially higher in obese adults, especially in those whose excessive fat is stored in the abdomen rather than in the hips. In fact, abdominal obesity is particularly dangerous because it leads to resistance to the actions of insulin, the hormone that regulates blood glucose. Insulin resistance

under 25) throughout life, more than 90,000 annual deaths from cancer could be prevented.

How Obesity Promotes Cancer
A variety of factors are thought to raise an obese person's risk of developing cancer in the first place and then of dying of cancer once it develops. The most apparent potential causes are related to inactivity and to a nutritionally inadequate diet. Additional underlying factors may include:

Acid reflux. Obesity, particularly abdominal fat, contributes to chronic acid reflux, which damages the lining of the lower esophagus and increases the risk of esophageal cancer.

High caloric intake. Consuming too many calories may promote tumor growth. For unknown reasons, long-term caloric restriction prevents cancer in laboratory animals that consume only 60% of their normal caloric intake. Accumulating evidence from human studies supports the cancer-protective effect of calorie restriction.

Carcinogens. Once in the body, cancer-causing agents tend to accumulate in body fat. Their subsequent release may stimulate tumor growth.

Diagnosis and treatment. Research suggests that obese individuals may be less likely to survive cancer because their cancers are more often diagnosed at a late stage. Late stage diagnosis may possibly occur because obese individuals are less likely to undergo routine cancer screenings, or screening methods may be less effective for detecting cancer in early stages than in the nonobese. Furthermore, certain cancer treatments may be less effective in obese individuals.

Gallstones. Obesity increases the risk of gallstone formation, which elevates the risk of developing gallbladder cancer.

Insulin and growth factors. Obesity increases blood levels of the hormone insulin (which lowers blood sugar) and insulin-related growth factors. Elevated levels of these compounds fuel cell division, and that may overstimulate cell proliferation and increase the risk of developing tumors of the breast (premenopausal), colon, prostate, and rectum.

Sex hormones. Excessive body fat appears to prompt the overproduction of the sex hormones estrogen and testosterone, which, in turn, are believed to trigger hormone-dependent cancers, including breast, prostate, and uterine tumors.

Questions Remain
While mounting evidence points to a significant link between excessive body weight and cancer, vital questions remain unanswered. Researchers have yet to uncover all of the exact causes underlying the obesity-cancer connection and the extent to which overweight and obesity may influence the biological course of various cancers and alter the chances of successful treatment. There is currently little scientific information regarding the relationship between BMI and the risk of certain malignancies, such as cancers of the blood. In addition, the location of excessive body fat may play a role in cancer development and survival. For instance, some findings indicate that abdominal obesity, in particular, is linked to malignancies of the colon, prostate, and rectum.

Furthermore, childhood obesity as well as weight changes during adulthood may affect cancer risk. Additional research is needed to fully determine the impact of obesity on cancer development and survival.

Recommendations and Weight Loss Strategies
To minimize cancer risk associated with excessive weight, experts recommend the tips listed below.

- Maintain a lifelong, healthy body weight, defined as a BMI under 25.
- Gain no more than 11 lbs. over a healthy body weight (a BMI under 25) during adulthood.
- Take off any excess weight. Aim for a gradual 1- to 2-lb. loss per week.
- Reduce caloric intake by limiting portion sizes and the consumption of calorie-dense foods.
- Eat a nutritionally balanced, wholesome diet rich in fruits, vegetables, and whole grains.
- Engage in one hour of moderate activity on most days of the week.
- Minimize acid reflux with dietary changes and, if necessary, medical treatment.
- Consult with your physician about routine cancer screenings.

results in elevated blood levels of insulin, which is associated with high triglycerides, low HDL cholesterol, high blood pressure, and increased CHD risk, a constellation of conditions called metabolic syndrome. (For more information on metabolic syndrome, see the feature on page 56.)

Metabolic Syndrome: A Cluster of Related Problems

Most people have never heard of this surprisingly common condition in which obesity plays a role.

For many years, physicians have recognized that elevated blood glucose levels, high blood pressure, obesity, and abnormal blood lipid levels tend to occur together in certain individuals. This cluster of symptoms—previously called the Deadly Quartet, syndrome X, or insulin resistance syndrome—is now commonly referred to as metabolic syndrome. Almost one in four American adults has metabolic syndrome, which increases the risk of diabetes, coronary heart disease, and strokes.

Diagnosis and Prevalence

In 2001, the National Cholesterol Education Program (sponsored by the National Heart, Lung, and Blood Institute) proposed the following criteria for the diagnosis of metabolic syndrome. A person needs to have at least three of the following five factors to be diagnosed with the condition:

- abdominal obesity (a waist circumference greater than 40 inches in men or 35 inches in women);
- triglyceride levels of 150 mg/dL or greater;
- high density lipoprotein (HDL) cholesterol levels of less than 40 mg/dL in men or 50 mg/dL in women;
- blood pressure of 130/85 mm Hg or higher, or taking an antihypertensive medication; or
- fasting blood glucose (sugar) levels of 110 mg/dL or greater.

While only 7% of men and women age 20 to 29 meet this definition of metabolic syndrome, the percentage rises to more than 40% of those age 60 and older. The condition is more common in Mexican Americans (32%) than in whites (24%) or blacks (22%).

Causes

Virtually all people with metabolic syndrome have insulin resistance, a decreased ability of the body's tissues to respond to insulin. Insulin enables cells to take up glucose from the blood for use as a source of energy. In an insulin-resistant person, cells do not respond adequately to the effects of insulin, and insufficient amounts of glucose enter the cells. As a result, the pancreas produces more insulin to help glucose move into the cells, and blood insulin levels rise. Eventually, the pancreas can no longer produce enough insulin to compensate for the insulin resistance, blood glucose levels rise, and diabetes develops.

Even before the onset of diabetes, however, people may have elevated blood pressure. Increased production of triglycerides by the liver can lead to abnormalities in blood lipid levels, including high triglycerides, low levels of HDL cholesterol, and increased levels of small, dense low density lipoprotein (LDL) particles (which are more likely to cause blood clots than larger LDL particles).

Exactly what causes insulin resistance is unclear. However, researchers do know that genetic factors, obesity, physical inactivity, diet, cigarette smoking, and older age each contribute to insulin resistance and therefore to metabolic syndrome. Other factors that make a person more likely to develop insulin resistance include a family history of diabetes in a first-degree relative (a parent or sibling), a personal history of

A recent report in the *Journal of the American College of Cardiology* further clarified the relationship between obesity and insulin resistance. Researchers measured insulin sensitivity in 314 individuals free from diabetes and hypertension and determined that the likelihood of insulin resistance rose in tandem with a rising body mass index (BMI). However, the BMI alone did not predict insulin resistance: About 20% of those with the syndrome had a normal weight (BMI less than 25), and some obese individuals (a BMI over 30) were not insulin resistant, indicating that other factors also play a role. For any given level of obesity, however, insulin-resistant individuals are at significantly greater risk for developing coronary artery disease than those with normal insulin sensitivity. In addition, this study determined that the risk factors most strongly asso-

gestational diabetes (diabetes during pregnancy), or polycystic ovary syndrome (a condition characterized by infrequent or absent menstruation, infertility, and excessive body hair).

Complications

Metabolic syndrome increases the risk of numerous complications. Because of its association with insulin resistance, people with metabolic syndrome are more likely to have type 2 diabetes. In turn, diabetes increases the risk of vision problems, kidney dysfunction, nerve problems, coronary heart disease, and strokes.

High blood pressure, high triglycerides, and low HDL cholesterol are all risk factors for atherosclerosis. Elevated insulin levels are also associated with an increased tendency for blood clot formation. As a result, people with metabolic syndrome have a greater incidence of all types of cardiovascular disease (including nonfatal and fatal heart attacks and strokes) and are at increased risk for premature death from any cause.

Treatment

Treatment of metabolic syndrome focuses on overcoming insulin resistance and correcting any associated abnormalities. The first step in treatment is lifestyle changes. The most important lifestyle change is weight loss through increased physical activity, decreased intake of calories (particularly simple carbohydrates), and increased fiber intake.

Physical activity aids in weight loss, improves responsiveness to insulin, increases HDL levels, and decreases blood pressure. An increase in activity need not be dramatic to achieve significant health benefits—even a half hour of brisk walking most days of the week will help.

Weight loss improves insulin sensitivity, reduces elevated insulin levels, and lowers the risk of developing type 2 diabetes. While reduced insulin resistance can occur with as little as a 5-lb. weight loss, better results are achieved with a 7% to 15% decrease in body weight. A diet rich in fiber-containing foods—such as fruits, vegetables, and whole grains—can help overcome insulin resistance. Smoking cessation can lessen insulin resistance and help to raise HDL cholesterol levels.

If lifestyle modifications do not correct the associated cardiovascular risk factors, medications can lower blood pressure and improve lipid levels. Thiazide-type diuretics are considered first-choice therapy for hypertension because they prevent heart attacks and strokes. ACE inhibitors are also a good for those with metabolic syndrome because they may reduce the risk of developing type 2 diabetes, in addition to lowering blood pressure. Some people with metabolic syndrome may require statins, which lower LDL cholesterol and raise HDL cholesterol levels. Niacin, gemfibrozil (Lopid), and fenofibrate (Lofibra, Tricor) can also raise HDL cholesterol and lower triglyceride levels.

Metformin (Glucophage) and the thiazolidinediones pioglitazone (Actos) and rosiglitazone (Avandia) are currently used to treat insulin resistance in people with type 2 diabetes. Also, according to a 2002 study in *The New England Journal of Medicine,* people at high risk for diabetes (those who are overweight and have elevated blood glucose levels) can prevent or delay the development of diabetes with lifestyle changes and, less markedly, with metformin. However, it is not yet clear whether these medications should be used to treat the insulin resistance that leads to metabolic syndrome.

ciated with insulin resistance were elevated triglyceride levels and low levels of HDL cholesterol.

Excess weight also increases the risk of gallbladder disease and places greater stress on the back, hips, and knees, which may aggravate arthritis. In addition, obesity can lead to mental anguish due to poor body image, social isolation, and social discrimination.

MEDICAL EVALUATION OF WEIGHT

Anyone who is over age 40 or has health problems should have a thorough medical evaluation prior to beginning a weight loss program. In addition, your physician may refer you to a nutritionist for an assessment of eating habits.

Medical History

The medical history will include the following:

Weight history. Your physician will determine how long you have been overweight, because obesity present since childhood may reflect a genetic predisposition and is often more difficult to treat than adult-onset obesity. Other questions may address dieting history: Have you tried a variety of diets? Is there a pattern of weight loss and gain (called weight cycling or "yo-yo" dieting)?

Medical history. Do you have any symptoms or history of obesity-related disorders (such as CHD, stroke, hypertension, cancer, or diabetes)? Are there any symptoms suggesting an endocrine cause of obesity, such as hypothyroidism?

Family history. Is obesity prevalent in your family? Is there a family history of any obesity-related disorders?

Medications. Drugs that can cause weight gain, increase appetite, or hinder weight loss include corticosteroids, progestins, tricyclic antidepressants, phenothiazines, lithium, sulfonylureas, thiazolidinediones, and insulin.

Depressive symptoms. Depression affects many overweight people, especially those who are severely obese. A thorough evaluation includes questions about mood to determine whether depression needs to be treated along with obesity.

Physical Examination

Blood pressure, height, weight, and waist circumference are measured. The physician will look for evidence of cardiovascular disease (diseases of the heart and blood vessels), osteoarthritis, and hypothyroidism or other hormonal conditions.

Obesity is often defined as weighing 20% or more above ideal body weight (which varies with height, age, and gender). This definition is somewhat misleading, however, since it is not the amount of excess weight, but the amount of excess adipose tissue—or body fat—that determines the threat to health. It is possible to be overweight without being obese, as in the case of a weight lifter who has built up muscle mass. Moreover, the distribution of body fat is an important predictor of health risk—fat stored in the abdominal area is more harmful than fat stored in the hips, thighs, and buttocks. The degree of obesity is also important; a mildly obese person is at less risk for developing obesity-related conditions than someone who is morbidly obese (a BMI of 40 or more).

In addition to height, age, and gender, a person's ideal weight depends on many factors, including body composition (the propor-

Are You Overweight?

Although most people rely on the bathroom scale to determine if they're overweight, a better way to find out if weight and distribution of body fat are unhealthy is to calculate body mass index (BMI) and waist circumference.

According to current national guidelines, overweight is defined as a BMI of 25 to 29.9 and obesity as a BMI of 30 and above. While BMI is a general assessment of body weight and disease risk, waist circumference provides an added and more specific measure of health risk because waist circumference estimates harmful abdominal fat. Even in normal weight people, an increased weight circumference is linked to an elevated health risk, especially for diabetes and cardiovascular disease. And in men and women who are overweight or obese, a high waist circumference increases the already greater risk of disease.

Body Mass Index
BMI is your body weight in kilograms divided by your squared height in meters. To calculate your BMI using pounds and inches, follow these simple steps:

1. Multiply your weight (in pounds) by 703.
2. Square your height (in inches) by multiplying the number by itself.
3. Divide the result of step 1 by the result of step 2.

Waist Circumference
To measure your waist circumference, wrap a tape measure around your waist at the level of the top of your hip bones; it should feel snug without compressing the skin. Measure after exhaling normally. A normal waist circumference is less than 40 inches in men and less than 35 inches in women.

tion of fat and muscle), body shape (where fat is deposited), and general health. The most accurate way to assess the degree of obesity is to measure the amount of body fat. Since this task is not easy to perform, doctors generally rely on surrogate measures, such as body mass index and waist circumference, or use height/weight tables.

The National Heart, Lung, and Blood Institute and the National Institute of Diabetes and Digestive and Kidney Diseases have issued guidelines on the identification, evaluation, and treatment of overweight and obesity. Body mass index and waist circumference were found to be most useful for determining the need for weight loss. The pros and cons of most methods of weight assessment are discussed below.

Height/weight tables. Height/weight tables are the most straightforward way to assess your weight, but there are drawbacks to relying solely on this method. The tables are not based on scientific calculations of ideal weight but instead are derived from height, weight, and mortality data of people seeking life insurance. Moreover, they do not take into account body composition; and, because the tables suggest weight goals that are difficult for most obese people to achieve or maintain, they often lead to frustration for people who are attempting to lose weight.

Body mass index (BMI). As the result of the difficulty in directly measuring the amount of body fat and the drawbacks of using height/weight tables alone, researchers have turned to a measurement called body mass index to define obesity and its severity. BMI is a measurement of your weight as it relates to your height (see the BMI calculation on page 59). BMI correlates strongly with the amount of body fat, though it does not measure it directly. Federal guidelines define overweight as a BMI from 25 to 29.9 and obesity as a BMI of 30 or greater. Morbid obesity is a BMI of 40 or greater.

Waist circumference. While BMI is a general assessment of body weight and disease risk, waist circumference provides an added and more specific measure of health risk because waist circumference indicates harmful abdominal fat. Research shows that the mortality rates and incidence of certain chronic diseases, such as diabetes and high blood pressure, are substantially higher in those with a disproportionate amount of body fat stored in the abdomen.

Fortunately, abdominal fat is often the first to go with weight loss. Typically, men are prone to fat deposition in the abdomen—developing what is commonly called a pot belly, beer belly, or apple shape—whereas women tend to accumulate fat around the hips, buttocks, and thighs, a distribution called a pear shape. Some researchers believe that women are naturally programmed to store fat in the lower body for use as an energy reserve during pregnancy and breast feeding. However, women are not immune to accumulating abdominal fat, and weight tends to be stored in a pattern typical to a particular individual (in other words, once a pear, always a pear).

Even in people of normal weight, an increased waist circumference may be linked to an elevated health risk. And in men and women who are overweight or obese, a large waist circumference increases the already elevated risk of disease. But people with a BMI of 35 or higher have a high risk of disease, regardless of their waist circumference. (See how to measure your waist circumference on page 59.)

Techniques for measuring body fat. Obesity is defined as fat stores exceeding 25% of total body weight for men or 30% for women. Direct measurement of the amount of body fat is the most accurate way to determine obesity-related health risk. A variety of methods can be used to estimate body fat, including underwater

NEW RESEARCH

Abdominal Obesity Linked to Ischemic Stroke Risk

Obesity is a risk factor for coronary heart disease, diabetes, and high blood pressure. Now, a study has firmly established a potent relationship between abdominal obesity and ischemic stroke.

Researchers determined the waist-to-hip ratio of 576 individuals who had suffered their first ischemic stroke and 1,142 patients who had never experienced a stroke. The waist-to-hip ratio is a measure of abdominal obesity.

Patients with high waist-to-hip ratios were three times more likely to have an ischemic stroke than those with low waist-to-hip ratios. The association held true for whites, blacks, and Hispanics and was greater in those less than 65 years of age. The link between ischemic stroke and abdominal obesity was just as strong as its association with blood pressure or diabetes found in previous studies.

Abdominal obesity, the researchers conclude, is a better predictor of ischemic stroke risk than BMI (body mass index), especially among younger people. They recommend that stroke prevention programs place greater emphasis on weight loss and preventing obesity.

STROKE
Volume 34, page 1586
July 2003

weighing (hydrodensitometry), dual-energy x-ray absorptiometry (DEXA), and bioelectrical impedance analysis (in which a small current of electricity is sent through the body). These techniques have the advantage of providing a more direct assessment of the proportion of total body weight that is fat. However, none of them is exact, some are expensive and not widely available, and all require trained personnel to administer them. Thus, they are not practical for general use.

Laboratory Tests

Blood will be drawn to measure total and HDL cholesterol, triglycerides, liver function, and blood glucose to screen for some of the complications of obesity. If a thyroid abnormality is suspected, thyroid stimulating hormone (TSH) is often measured.

LIFESTYLE TREATMENTS FOR WEIGHT LOSS

Successful weight loss requires a three-pronged approach: changing behavior patterns, making dietary adjustments, and increasing physical activity. Culled from medical research, the following guidelines incorporate strategies employed by people who have lost weight and kept it off. Use them to construct a weight loss program on your own or as an adjunct to medical or surgical treatments.

Behavioral Modification

An ability to alter lifelong attitudes toward diet and exercise may ultimately be the key to successful weight management: You must be motivated enough to change habits not for a few weeks or months, but for a lifetime. The importance of this resolve cannot be underestimated.

The desire to lose weight must come from within, rather than from external pressures. A person who wants to shed 20 lbs. to please a spouse is not likely to be as motivated, or as successful, as someone whose goal is to improve health or increase self-esteem. Choosing the right time to start a weight-loss program is also important. People under stress or pressure may not be able to devote the considerable attention and effort required to make lifestyle changes.

If you are motivated and ready to lose weight, the following guidelines will help.

1. Set realistic goals. Remember that weight tables give estimates of ideal weights; you can probably be healthy at weights above "ideal" if you have a nutritious diet and exercise. Instead of attempting to lose a specific number of pounds, make it your goal to adopt

Emotional Strategies for Weight Loss

To lose weight and maintain a healthy weight permanently, experts suggest the following strategies to boost your motivation to eat well and exercise regularly:

- Learn to manage stress, which can trigger poor eating habits. Adopt coping strategies such as meditation and deep breathing exercises.
- Identify and control triggers that encourage overeating and inactivity. For example, keep junk food out of the house; or, if it is in the house, do not leave it in plain sight. Plan a social event around physical activity, instead of food.
- Reward positive behavior. Whether it is monetary or verbal, from yourself or a friend, a reward for good eating and exercise habits reinforces the positive behavior.
- Change self-defeating thoughts. A negative internal dialogue can easily undermine weight loss efforts, so as often as possible consciously replace negative thoughts and feelings with more constructive, optimistic ones. For instance, instead of criticizing yourself for eating junk food for breakfast, focus on a plan to eat better for the rest of the day.
- Keep a journal to monitor eating and exercise habits. For example, record the amount and caloric value of food that you eat, along with the time, place, and any feelings associated with the situation.
- Assemble a strong social network for support. Friends, family, and colleagues can offer enthusiasm and inspiration that boost weight loss incentive.
- Seek professional nutrition counseling, if necessary. According to 2003 recommendations from the U.S. Preventive Task Services Task Force, intensive diet counseling can particularly help adults at risk for chronic diseases, such as high cholesterol or high blood pressure. Diet counseling, defined as several 30-minute sessions with a primary care physician or registered dietitian, has been shown to help at-risk adults eat less fat and more fruits and vegetables.

healthier eating and exercise habits. If you are obese and feel compelled to set a weight goal, losing 10% to 15% of your current body weight is a realistic objective. The good news is that evidence shows that weight loss of as little as 5% to 10% of body weight can significantly improve risk factors such as blood pressure and blood glucose. The safest rate of weight loss is ½ to 2 lbs. a week.

2. Seek support from family and friends. People who receive social support are more successful in changing their behaviors. Ask family and friends for help, whether this means keeping high-fat foods out of the house or relieving you of some chore so that you have time to exercise. It will be easier to stick to your new eating plan if everyone in the household eats the same types of foods. (A low-fat diet that includes plenty of fruits, vegetables, and grains will benefit your family's health even if they do not need to lose weight.) You may be more motivated to exercise if you work out with a friend or family member.

3. Make changes gradually. Trying to make many changes quickly can leave you feeling overwhelmed and frustrated. Instead, ease into exercise; do not overdo it. Incorporate low-fat eating in stages. For example, if you typically drink whole milk, switch to reduced-fat (2%) milk, then to low-fat (1%), and then to fat-free milk. With this approach, you will not notice the difference in taste as much. In fact, your taste preferences will actually change—the once-favored high-fat foods will start tasting too rich and greasy after you have eaten low-fat foods for a while. Another tactic is to switch to low-fat foods one meal at a time. For example, concentrate on eating a low-fat breakfast for one week, add lunch the next week, and then dinner the third week.

4. Eat slowly. Many people consume more calories than needed to satisfy their hunger because they eat too quickly. Since it takes about 20 minutes for the brain to recognize that the stomach is full, slowing down helps you feel satisfied on less food. Moreover, eating slowly allows you to better appreciate the flavors and textures of your food.

5. Eat three meals a day, plus snacks. Skipping meals is counterproductive, as is severely reducing food intake, since such strict changes are impossible to maintain and are ultimately unhealthy. People who restrict their eating habits too rigorously often have an "all or nothing" approach: Once they go off their diet, they tend to abandon all efforts and find it difficult to return to healthy eating. In addition, eating the bulk of your calories at one sitting may impair metabolism. You will be more successful in the long run if you allow yourself to eat when you are hungry, eat enough nutritious low-fat food to satisfy that hunger, and spread your calorie intake over the course of the day.

6. Plan for exercise. Choose activities that are convenient and enjoyable for you to do on a regular basis, and then treat exercise like any other appointment—set a time and jot it down in your date book. Many people find it easier to exercise first thing in the morning, before the demands of the day interfere, but others find lunchtime or right after work more convenient.

7. Record your progress. Start a food diary and exercise log to keep track of your accomplishments. Keeping such detailed diaries may seem cumbersome, but they can help you stay motivated, and reviewing the entries can reveal any problem areas. In addition, the information can help facilitate treatment by your nutritionist or doctor.

8. Evaluate your relationship to food. Behavioral and emotional cues frequently trigger an inappropriate desire to eat. The most common cues are habit, stress, boredom, sadness, anxiety, loneliness, and the use of food as a reward. Many people also relate food to love or care and derive comfort from it. Although eating may appear to soothe uncomfortable feelings, its effect is temporary at best and ultimately does not solve any problems. In fact, it may distract you from focusing on the real issues.

9. Recall your accomplishments. Over your lifetime you have probably been successful in tackling many difficult tasks—quitting smoking, learning a new skill, or advancing in the workplace, for example. Reminding yourself of past achievements can help you feel more confident about making the changes that will lead to weight loss.

10. Don't try to be perfect. While losing weight requires significant changes in eating and exercise habits, not every high-calorie food must be banished forever, and you need not exercise vigorously every day. High-calorie foods can be eaten once in a while without hindering weight loss. On days when you have a candy bar, for example, compensate for the extra fat and calories by eliminating a few calories and grams of fat from your diet over the next few days. And "cravings" for high-calorie foods can often be satisfied by small tastes—a piece of chocolate rather than a whole candy bar. It is also acceptable to miss an exercise session. On days when you do not feel like doing formal exercise, take a brisk walk instead. (Remember that calories are also burned during nonexercise activities, such as housework. See "Burning Calories with Everyday Activities" on page 72.)

Diet

To determine how many calories you should eat per day, first calculate the number of calories needed to maintain your current weight—roughly 15 calories per pound of body weight in a moderately active person (someone who gets at least 30 minutes of moderate to intense physical activity every day). For example, a moderately active 150-lb. person who consumes 2,250 calories per day will neither gain nor lose weight. A completely sedentary person may require just 12 calories per pound to maintain weight.

A pound of body fat contains 3,500 calories. To lose one to two pounds per week—a gradual and safe rate of weight loss—you must eat 500 to 1,000 fewer calories per day than what is needed to maintain your weight. (The calorie cutback need not be so severe if you also begin to exercise regularly.) Calorie intake should not drop below 1,200 per day in women or 1,500 per day in men (unless the diet is medically supervised and you are taking a vitamin/mineral supplement), since it would be difficult to get all the nutrients you need.

While reducing calorie intake is essential for losing weight, focusing on calories per se may leave people feeling hungry and frustrated unless the overall composition of the diet is also considered. Replacing dietary fat with complex carbohydrates automatically lowers calorie intake, while allowing a satisfying volume of food. For any given number of calories, you can eat a much larger amount of food on a low-fat diet than on a high-fat diet. The reason for this is simple: Gram for gram, fat contains more than twice as many calories as carbohydrates or protein: nine versus four calories. Fatty foods also contain less water and fiber—substances that help make a food more filling—than foods high in complex carbohydrates. But, all too often, people reduce their intake of fat and instead consume an equal or greater amount of calories in the form of simple carbohydrates.

There are other reasons to reduce the fat content of your diet. Some evidence suggests that a prolonged high-fat diet may trigger an upward adjustment in the body's set point. In addition, fewer calories are burned when dietary fat is converted into body fat than when carbohydrates or protein are converted into fat. Moreover, a low-fat diet can help to lower blood cholesterol levels and may reduce the risk of colon and prostate cancer. And not just the amount, but the type of fat you eat affects your health risks: Saturated fats, found in animal products like meat and cheese, are more harmful than monounsaturated or polyunsaturated fats.

Once you decide on an appropriate calorie intake, you need to determine the amount of total fat you should eat. Most experts now recommend that a diet should derive no more than 35% of its calories from fat (even when substituting monounsaturated for saturated fats). Most people should not reduce fat intake to less than 20% of calories, and the American Heart Association (AHA) cautions against cutting fat below 15% for certain groups of people (older adults, for example) owing to concerns over malnutrition and a possible negative effect on blood lipids. The following guidelines will help you adopt a low-fat, high-complex-carbohydrate diet.

1. Eat mostly fruits, vegetables, legumes, and grains. These foods are naturally low in fat and high in fiber. (Fiber provides bulk, which helps to fill you up without adding calories.) The wide variety of these foods provides different textures and flavors, so you will not feel bored or deprived.

2. Do not add fat during cooking. Avoid sautéing foods in butter

NEW RESEARCH

Obesity Increases the Risk of Reflux

People who are obese, especially women, have an increased risk of developing gastroesophageal reflux symptoms like heartburn and regurgitation.

According to a new study, severely obese men (i.e., a BMI greater than 35) have a three times greater risk of reflux symptoms than men with a normal body mass (a BMI of less than 25). Severely obese women have six times the risk of reflux symptoms. Also, severely obese premenopausal women are much more likely to have reflux symptoms than severely obese postmenopausal women, suggesting that female sex hormones may play a role in the relationship between obesity and reflux.

These results were based on a 1995 to 1997 survey of 65,363 Norwegians. Many of these individuals also participated in an earlier (1984 to 1986) survey of 74,599 Norwegians. People who lost weight between the first and second survey were less likely to have reflux symptoms at the second survey than those who didn't lose weight, indicating that weight loss can reduce the risk of reflux.

Obese premenopausal women are likely to have higher levels of active estrogen, which the researchers hypothesize may increase the synthesis of nitric oxide. Nitric oxide might lead to reflux by relaxing the smooth muscle in the lower esophageal sphincter, potentially leading to reflux.

JOURNAL OF THE AMERICAN MEDICAL ASSOCIATION
Volume 290, page 66
July 2, 2003

Comparing Artificial Sweeteners

Here is the latest research on the five sugar substitutes now on the market.

Americans, in a continuing quest for low-calorie diets, are buying artificially sweetened foods (such as soft drinks, salad dressings, yogurt, and baked goods) in ever-increasing numbers. A recent survey shows that approximately 163 million Americans regularly consume reduced-calorie, sugar-free products. But are these food items safe? Here's the latest research on the five sugar substitutes currently approved by the U.S. Food and Drug Administration (FDA): saccharin, aspartame, acesulfame potassium, sucralose, and neotame.

Health Professionals Approve . . . With Caveats

Many health organizations, such as the American Heart Association and the American Diabetes Association, approve of the use of artificial sweeteners for weight reduction, as long as they are part of an overall weight control program that includes exercise and other dietary measures. However, many artificially sweetened foods and beverages are not nutritious, and some people fill up on them rather than on healthful foods. In addition, their use may encourage people to maintain a preference for sweet foods that can lead to overindulgence and weight gain, the very problem artificial sweeteners are aimed at correcting.

While questions regarding the safety of some of these artificial sweeteners have arisen over the years, current evidence indicates that they are all safe. Before an artificial sweetener is deemed safe and made available to consumers, it must undergo rigorous investigation by the FDA. The FDA regularly monitors safety information on artificial sweeteners and may take action to protect the public if credible scientific evidence indicates a safety problem.

A Closer Look

The following is an overview of the five artificial sweeteners currently approved by the FDA.

Saccharin. Discovered in 1879, saccharin (Sweet 'N Low) is the oldest of the artificial sweeteners. Saccharin was used during both world wars to help compensate for sugar shortages. Three hundred times sweeter than sugar, saccharin is popular as a tabletop sweetener in restaurants, where it is available in single-serving packets.

Saccharin has been the subject of ongoing controversy: Large amounts of saccharin can cause bladder cancer in rats, and it was suspected of causing cancer in humans, though studies have not supported this association. In 1977, the FDA declared that it was going to prohibit saccharin use, on the basis of animal studies. Instead, a warning label was issued for the product stating, "use of this product may be hazardous to your health ... [and] it has been determined to cause cancer in laboratory animals."

Congress passed a moratorium preventing an FDA-proposed saccharin ban, and in 1991 the FDA formally withdrew its 1977 proposal to ban the use of saccharin while additional safety studies were conducted. In 2000, a bill was signed by the Presi-

or oil. Use nonstick pans; coat them lightly with cooking spray if necessary, or try using broth, wine, fruit juice or even water for sautéing. Bake, broil, steam, or roast foods instead of frying them.

3. Choose lean cuts of meat and poultry. Meat and poultry are rich in nutrients and good sources of high-quality protein, but they can also contain a lot of fat. Top round, eye of round, and round are the leanest cuts of beef; tenderloin, top loin, and lean ham are the leanest pork cuts; and light-meat chicken and turkey are leaner than dark meat. Completely trim all external fat from meat before cooking. Do not eat poultry skin—it contains a lot of fat. But you can leave it on during roasting or baking to help keep the meat moist and tender; just be sure you do not cook the poultry with other ingredients, such as potatoes, that could absorb the fat released

dent to remove the warning label on saccharin-sweetened products. The FDA supported the repeal of the warning label, and other government researchers, scientists, and industry have agreed that saccharin is indeed safe for human use.

Aspartame. Approved by the FDA in 1981, aspartame (NutraSweet, Equal) is 180 to 200 times sweeter than sugar. As with saccharin, aspartame has been the subject of intense controversy. For example, anecdotal reports assert that the consumption of aspartame can lead to a range of adverse reactions, including headaches, tumors, seizures, panic attacks, hyperactivity, and multiple sclerosis. There is no conclusive scientific evidence, however, to support these claims.

It is ironic that aspartame is frequently the subject of these allegations because, according to the FDA, aspartame is the most thoroughly tested and widely studied food additive that the agency has ever approved. In fact, more than 100 studies verify that aspartame is safe for the general population. Aspartame's only proven danger is for people with phenylketonuria, a rare genetic disorder. Currently, more than 100 million people around the world consume aspartame-containing products.

Acesulfame potassium. First approved by the FDA in 1988, acesulfame potassium (Sunett, Sweet One) is about 200 times sweeter than sugar. Because it is so sweet, it is often blended with other artificial sweeteners, such as aspartame, to produce a more sugar-like taste. Acesulfame potassium (called acesulfame-k on food labels) is approved for use in baked goods, frozen desserts, candies (including breath mints, cough drops, and lozenges), and beverages. It is also currently used in thousands of foods, beverages, and oral hygiene and pharmaceutical products in about 90 countries.

Sucralose. In 1998, the FDA approved sucralose (Splenda) as a tabletop sweetener and for use in products such as baked goods, nonalcoholic beverages, chewing gum, frozen dairy desserts, fruit juices, and gelatins. Sucralose is 600 times sweeter than sugar. Sucralose is the only artificial sweetener made from sugar. It has no calories and retains its sweetness over a wide range of temperatures and storage conditions.

Neotame. Approved by the FDA in July 2002, neotame is sweeter than other artificial sweeteners—7,000 to 13,000 times sweeter than sugar—and is approximately 30 to 40 times sweeter than aspartame. Neotame is found in numerous processed foods and can be used as a tabletop sweetener.

Cooking With Sugar Substitutes

Owing to their stability at high temperatures, most sugar substitutes don't degrade when exposed to heat and are suitable for use in home cooking and baking. Aspartame, however, tends to lose sweetness when baked at high temperatures, though it can be added during the last few minutes of heating or cooking.

When you substitute an artificial sweetener for sugar in a recipe, you will need to experiment with small amounts of the sugar substitute (since they are all so much sweeter than sugar) to get the right amount of sweetness. Make sure to read labels carefully to achieve the best results.

from the skin as it cooks. Limit portion sizes to 3 oz.—about the size of the palm of your hand or a deck of cards—and round out the meal with plenty of grains and vegetables.

4. Switch to low-fat or fat-free dairy products. Whole milk and cheeses can contain more fat than meat does. For example, 1 oz. of cheddar has the same amount of fat as a 6-oz. chicken breast or a 3½-oz. sirloin. But do not eliminate dairy products: They are an important source of calcium and protein. Instead, select fat-free milk and fat-free yogurt, along with limited amounts of reduced-fat or part-skim cheeses.

5. Read food labels. The nutrition labels that are required on all packaged foods provide important information about their calorie and fat content, which makes it easy to compare brands.

Serving sizes are arbitrary, however, so be sure to compare equal portions.

6. Experiment with reduced-fat, low-fat, and fat-free versions of foods. From fat-free milk to reduced-fat salad dressing and cream cheese, these foods can help you cut fat from your diet. Just because a food is low in fat does not mean you can eat unlimited quantities, however, since it can still provide a lot of calories. For example, some fat-free cakes and cookies contain as many—or more—calories than the regular versions because manufacturers add extra sugar to compensate for flavor lost when fat is removed.

7. Use fat substitutes judiciously. While fat substitutes definitely reduce the number of calories consumed from fat and saturated fat, their impact on total caloric intake and body weight, as well as general health in the long term, is uncertain. And one fat substitute, olestra—used in some chips and crackers—inhibits the absorption of fat-soluble nutrients. Vitamins A, D, E, and K are added to products to offset this effect.

8. Watch out for hidden fats. It is easy to overlook the fat and calories contributed by toppings such as margarine, cream sauce, mayonnaise, salad dressings, peanut butter, sour cream, and cheese. Limit the amounts of these items; choose low-fat versions (such as nonfat sour cream or mayonnaise); or find substitutes (for example, tomato sauce instead of cream sauce on pasta).

9. Consider the calories in beverages. Although regular soda, fruit juices, and alcoholic beverages are fat free, they contain a significant number of calories. And, with the exception of citrus juices, these beverages are not a good source of vitamins and minerals. Choose calorie-free beverages—water or seltzer, and moderate amounts of coffee and tea—most of the time. Limit your alcohol intake: Try nonalcoholic beer (which has fewer calories than regular beer) or mix wine with seltzer for a lower-calorie wine spritzer. Lessen the calories in fruit juices by mixing them with seltzer, or eat the fruit instead—it has fewer calories than the juice and it satisfies hunger better because of its fiber.

10. Control portion sizes. While fat consumption has dropped in the past 20 years in the United States, serving sizes and total calorie consumption have increased. Americans tend to eat large portions of food, especially meat, and what many people think of as a serving is usually more than the amount that is listed in nutrition tables and on food labels. For example, a serving of breakfast cereal is about one cup, but many people fill their bowls with much more than that. And according to recent research, almost all

NEW RESEARCH

Fat Intake, Excess Weight Increase Risk of Alzheimer's

People with high intakes of unhealthy fats and overweight women are at increased risk of Alzheimer's disease, according to two new reports.

The first report looked at 815 people, age 65 to 94, from Chicago. Those with the highest intakes of saturated fat or trans fatty acids developed Alzheimer's twice as often over a four-year period than people with the lowest intake of these fats. On the other hand, intakes of omega-6 polyunsaturated fats (found in fish, nuts, seeds, and corn, soy, and safflower oils) and monounsaturated fat (found in olive and canola oils, almonds, and avocados) were linked to a lower Alzheimer's risk.

The second report evaluated 392 Swedes. Women with a slightly higher BMI at age 70 had a greater likelihood of developing Alzheimer's disease during 18 years of follow-up than women with a lower BMI. No relationship was seen between BMI and dementia in men, possibly because overweight men may not live long enough to develop dementia.

Together, these studies suggest that diet, particularly fat intake, and body weight may play a significant role in the likelihood of developing Alzheimer's disease.

ARCHIVES OF NEUROLOGY
Volume 60, page 194
February 2003

ARCHIVES OF INTERNAL MEDICINE
Volume 163, page 1,524
July 14, 2003

foods and beverages currently sold in the United States are excessive in size and dramatically increased from their original sizes. Hamburgers, french fries, and sodas are two to five times larger than they used to be in the 1970s. In addition, the average American eats about four restaurant meals a week; and studies show that most restaurant meals are not only larger in size than home-cooked meals, but they are also higher in calories, saturated fat, and sodium while being lower in fiber and calcium. Experts estimate that the dramatic increase in portion sizes could add 15 lbs. a year to the average person. And although the public has been educated about the fat in their diets, they may not realize that consuming the extra calories in super-sized portions can lead to weight gain.

To get an accurate picture of the amount of food you normally eat, serve yourself a typical portion, then use a measuring cup, measuring spoons, or a food scale to measure or weigh the food. Next, try serving yourself a smaller portion, eat it slowly, and see if your hunger is satisfied. (Keep in mind that you do not need to feel stuffed to satisfy your hunger.) You can dispense with weighing and measuring food once you become accustomed to estimating smaller portion sizes.

Fad Diets

Popular "fad" diets have been around for decades and are appealing because they often result in rapid, seemingly effortless weight loss, at least initially, owing to loss of body fluids. Recently, there has been an enormous resurgence in the popularity of low-carbohydrate (high-protein) diets. Such diets promote the same basic idea that was put forth in the 1960s: Eat high-protein foods (such as meat and eggs) and restrict carbohydrate-rich foods (such as potatoes, pasta, fruits, and certain vegetables).

Once relegated to the realm of quackery, these diets are being advocated because carbohydrates are thought to promote weight gain by increasing the body's production of insulin, which speeds up the conversion of food to body fat. Proponents of low-carbohydrate diets also claim that carbohydrates are less filling than other foods, causing people to consume more calories in an effort to satisfy their hunger. Furthermore, in some people, a low-fat, high-carbohydrate diet has been shown to raise triglyceride levels and lower HDL cholesterol levels—two components of metabolic syndrome, a cluster of conditions that can lead to heart disease and type 2 diabetes.

High-protein diets are being taken seriously by some researchers who concede that people can lose weight on them. In one study conducted at Duke University Medical Center, overweight people who were placed on a very-low-carbohydrate diet program achieved and maintained weight loss during a six-month period. Other studies are under way to investigate how these diets work.

However, several specific health concerns are associated with a diet that places such a heavy emphasis on the consumption of protein and the restriction of carbohydrate. Consuming too much protein imposes certain health risks. An inordinate intake of protein places extra stress on the liver and kidneys because they have to metabolize and excrete more than normal amounts of waste products. Kidney stones can be caused or aggravated by the high uric acid levels created by high-protein foods. And for those who have diabetes or kidney disease, high-protein diets can speed the progression of kidney disease, even if the diet is followed for a short time. Furthermore, some studies suggest that eating too much protein causes excessive calcium loss, which can contribute to osteoporosis.

Restricting carbohydrate intake is unhealthy as well. Drastically reducing carbohydrate consumption increases the metabolism of fatty acids and causes ketosis. This condition results when excessive amounts of acidic substances known as ketone bodies are released into the bloodstream. Ketosis can be dangerous for people with known or unrecognized heart disease, diabetes, or kidney problems. In addition, restricting carbohydrates can lead to vitamin and mineral deficiencies. Healthful, carbohydrate-rich foods, such as whole grains, fruits, and vegetables, provide essential nutrients as well as fiber and phytochemicals that work together to help prevent disease and promote good health. In fact, one of the basic underlying problems with most high-protein diets is their failure to promote a balanced diet and to teach long-term healthful eating habits.

High-protein, low-carbohydrate diets are best used selectively on a short-term basis, if at all, and under medical supervision. The many limitations and risks associated with high-protein diets raise important questions about their long-term safety and effectiveness. In fact, a 2003 advisory by the American College of Preventive Medicine (ACPM) states that there is currently little evidence to support the safety and effectiveness of popular diets that promote unlimited consumption of protein or fat. Nutrition experts maintain that the hallmarks of a healthy weight-loss diet are balance, flexibility, an emphasis on variety, and an ability to accommodate people with diverse needs and food preferences.

Exercise

Exercise is a valuable element in a weight loss program, but exercise alone results in only modest weight loss, and at a slower rate than calorie restriction. Studies have shown that combining exercise with diet results in greater loss of weight and body fat than dieting alone and is associated with a greater likelihood of maintaining weight loss. And adding exercise to calorie restriction makes the dietary changes easier because they need not be as drastic. It is easy to see why this is so. To lose one pound per week requires a deficit of about 500 calories a day. By adding a half hour of moderate to vigorous exercise per day (enough to burn 250 calories), you reduce the dietary restriction to a more manageable 250 calories per day.

Engage in activities that involve stretching, balance, aerobic exercise, and strength training. These types of exercise are generally recommended for older adults because they are low impact and help maintain overall strength, lower blood pressure, and strengthen bones. Exercise—especially strength training—helps to maintain muscle mass. Because muscle weighs more than fat, a person who exercises with strength training and cuts calories may lose less weight than one who only cuts calories, but the exerciser will lose more body fat.

The effect of exercise is cumulative. For example, while it takes about nine hours of walking at a normal pace for a 175-lb. person to burn 3,500 calories, the walking does not have to be completed all at once. You can achieve the same calorie deficit if you walk for half an hour each day for 18 days, or 45 minutes for 12 days, or an hour for 9 days. Even if you alternate days or work out only three times a week, you can still burn the same number of calories. You can even break up an exercise session into segments: For example, a 10-minute walk in the morning, 10 minutes at lunch, and 10 minutes in the evening still burn the same number of calories as a single 30-minute walk.

If you choose to use a personal trainer (either at home or at a gym), seek out a trainer who is properly qualified. A qualified trainer will have a bachelor's degree in exercise science or physical education or will be certified by the American College of Sports Medicine or the National Strength and Conditioning Association.

Start an exercise program gradually. Pushing too hard at the start may quickly cause frustration and the desire to quit. Trying to do too much, too soon may also lead to muscle strain and soreness, or even injury. Instead, increase your exercise level in the stages

NEW RESEARCH

Watching TV Linked to Obesity, Diabetes

People who watch large amounts of television increase their risk of becoming obese and developing diabetes, regardless of how much they exercise.

Doctors from Harvard found that every two hours a day spent watching television increased the risk of obesity by 23% and diabetes by 14%, independent of exercise levels. However, for every two hours a day spent walking or standing at home in activities like housework, the risks decreased by 9% for obesity and by 12% for diabetes.

The study involved data from 68,497 women who were followed for six years while participating in the Nurses' Health Study.

The authors of the report concluded that watching fewer than 10 hours of television per week and walking briskly for 30 or more minutes per day could prevent 30% and 43% of new cases of obesity and type 2 diabetes, respectively.

Television watching may lead to obesity, and therefore diabetes, because people tend to eat more food (especially unhealthy foods) while watching television than during other sedentary activities.

JOURNAL OF THE AMERICAN MEDICAL ASSOCIATION
Volume 289, page 1785
April 9, 2003

Burning Calories With Everyday Activities

The Surgeon General recommends a minimum of 30 minutes, or 150 calories' worth, of moderate-intensity physical activity at least five days a week. This is the amount needed to reap the general health benefits of exercise, including the prevention of diabetes and heart disease. For substantial weight loss, however, 30 minutes is not enough; experts at the Institute of Medicine recommend 60 minutes, or 300 calories' worth, of moderate activity each day.

The Centers for Disease Control and Prevention define moderate-intensity exercise as activity that burns approximately 3½ to 7 calories per minute, or about 150 calories in 30 minutes. You can burn those 150 calories by doing normal household chores, as well as by doing specific exercises. In addition, the same benefits can be achieved through a variety of activities: whether you run 1½ to 1¾ miles in 15 minutes or walk that distance in 35 minutes, you still burn the same 150 calories.

To fit 30 to 60 minutes of moderate activity into your weekly schedule and to continue with a routine, select activities that you enjoy, start gradually, and set aside the same time of day to exercise. Before embarking on any exercise program, be sure to first consult with your physician for recommendations, particularly if you are over age 50.

From least to most vigorous, moderate activities that burn 150 calories include:

- Washing and waxing a car for 45 to 60 minutes
- Gardening for 30 to 45 minutes
- Bicycling 5 miles in 30 minutes
- Raking leaves for 30 minutes
- Walking 2 miles in 30 minutes
- Swimming laps for 20 minutes
- Running 1½ miles for 15 minutes
- Shoveling snow for 15 minutes
- Walking up stairs for 15 minutes

described below. It is also important to make sure your exercise plan suits your lifestyle. For example, if you are a morning person, select that time to exercise.

And remember that sedentary people over the age of 50 should consult their doctor before starting any vigorous exercise program.

1. Increase your amount of everyday physical activity. The conveniences of modern life have made it easy to become sedentary. Look for ways to counteract the effects of these conveniences: for example, walk rather than drive, or take the stairs rather than an elevator or escalator. When doing errands or shopping, park some distance from your destination and walk the rest of the way. If you take public transportation, get off a few stops early and walk.

Walking up stairs can be a strenuous activity because you lift the full weight of your body with every step. Start slowly—begin by walking down flights of stairs, then start to walk up a flight or two at a time. Gradually increase the number of flights you climb at one time.

2. Add a formal walking program. Walking is appealing because it can be done anywhere, requires no special equipment (other than a supportive pair of shoes), and almost anyone can do it. Set your own pace: You expend approximately the same number of calories during an hour of slow walking as in half an hour of brisk walking. Start by walking for half an hour, three times a week. Once you become comfortable with this level of activity, walk for the same length of time five days a week. Next, gradually increase the duration of your walking to 40 minutes, then 50 minutes, and ultimately 1 hour. As you become more physically fit, you will be able to walk faster and go farther—and thus burn more calories in a given period of time.

3. Vary your activities. If you enjoy walking, make it the foundation of your exercise program. To prevent boredom, and also to work different muscle groups, choose other activities to substitute for walking on some days. Good choices include aerobic dance classes, bicycling, line dancing, or swimming. Swimming is a particularly good activity for older people who may have joint pain from arthritis. The buoyancy of the water lessens the strain on joints. Tennis and golf (provided you walk the course) can also burn calories. The most important rule, however, is to engage in activities that are enjoyable and convenient to do regularly.

4. Start a weight-training program. Working a muscle against resistance increases muscle size and strength. Because muscle takes up about 20% less space than fat, building muscle results in a leaner physique. In addition, having more muscle increases your metabolism, because it requires more energy to maintain muscle than fat tissue. You do not have to become a body builder or lift heavy weights to get the benefits. Working the major muscle groups—chest, arms, legs, and back—with light weights, two to three times a week, is sufficient. If you do not lose weight despite strength training, remember that you want to reduce body fat but not necessarily body weight, since muscle is denser and weighs more than fat.

MEDICAL AND SURGICAL TREATMENTS FOR OBESITY

Because the following treatments can be demanding for the patient and carry the risk of adverse side effects, they are appropriate only for people who are severely obese—especially those with, or at high risk for, medical conditions that may be improved with weight loss.

Very-Low-Calorie and Low-Calorie Diets

The term very-low-calorie diet (VLCD) is used to describe diets supplying fewer than 800 calories a day. Typically, patients must replace food with a powdered supplement that is combined with a non-caloric liquid (water or diet soda). To prevent deficiencies, the supplement is primarily made of high-quality protein derived from milk, eggs, or soy, along with a small amount of carbohydrates, minimal fat, and added vitamins and minerals. The high protein content of these diets is essential to help preserve muscle mass when calorie intake is so low. Recently, many centers modified their VLCD formulas to contain more calories. Studies have shown that weight loss is about as good on 800 as on 400 to 500 calories a day, and there are probably fewer risks. The term low-calorie diet (LCD) is used to describe diets that supply at least 800 calories per day to slightly below the person's daily caloric expenditure. So for a person needing 2,000 calories per day, a VLCD is up to 799 calories and an LCD is 800 to 1,999 calories. (Although a program may be referred to as a low-calorie diet, or LCD, we will use VLCD to describe both types, except where the protocols differ.)

Typically lasting 12 to 16 weeks, VLCDs require close medical supervision and are usually administered by weight loss clinics or hospitals. Programs should include regular medical monitoring; behavioral counseling to help you adjust to the diet; and instruction for changing eating patterns once food is reintroduced. Programs may also provide classes and support groups; many place a great emphasis on exercise. Once the VLCD phase is completed, food is slowly reintroduced over 2 to 10 weeks. The cost of participation is around $2,000 to $3,000. Few insurance companies cover this cost. If they do, it is usually covered only if the program is used to help treat a complication of severe obesity.

VLCDs are appropriate for people with a BMI of 35 or higher who have been unable to lose weight with conventional diet and exercise. LCDs are appropriate for individuals with a BMI between 30 and 34.9, especially for those who have coexisting conditions, such as type 2 diabetes, hypertension, high triglycerides, low HDL cholesterol, sleep apnea, or osteoarthritis.

Contraindications to VLCDs include a recent heart attack or stroke, heart rhythm abnormalities (arrhythmias), angina, liver or kidney disease, or type 1 diabetes. However, insulin-treated, obese patients with type 2 diabetes can benefit from VLCDs. For people who can stay on them, VLCDs produce dramatic reductions in weight. On average, participants lose 2.5 to 4 lbs. per week, at a rate that tends to slow as the duration of the VLCD increases to months.

Adding exercise to the program may enhance weight loss. Within three weeks, VLCDs often help lower blood pressure and cholesterol and triglyceride levels. In addition, glycemic control also improves.

Despite the dramatic success possible with VLCDs, they are not a panacea. About 25% of people who start a VLCD cannot adhere to the strict regimen and drop out of the program. Most of those who do complete treatment regain large amounts of weight within a year or two, typically reaching pretreatment weight within five years. In this way, VLCDs are no different from other diets. Most people can stick with dietary restrictions for a limited period of time. VLCDs may be even easier to follow than low-calorie diets that contain real food, because predetermined meals and controlled portion sizes help you to resist temptations.

However, you must learn to overcome the eating and behavioral patterns that contributed to your obesity in the first place—and you ultimately must make daily food choices on your own. As a result, VLCD programs are worthless without detailed attention to long-term maintenance. In one study, patients participated in a VLCD program with intensive behavioral training that included instructions on self-monitoring of eating behavior, guidelines for increasing physical activity, and techniques for counteracting relapse. The behavioral training continued even after the VLCD was finished and the patients returned to eating food. In six months, the patients lost an average of 45 lbs. One year later, they had regained only an average of 5 lbs.

In general, VLCDs are safe when medically supervised. Early side effects of hunger, fatigue, and light-headedness usually subside within two weeks. People who cannot tolerate milk products may react to a dairy-based formula. Later on, dieters may note constipation and intolerance to cold, and the risk of gallstones is increased.

Medications

Whether the treatment of obesity requires medication is a decision that must be made on a case-by-case basis. Drug therapy was never intended to be anything but a last-choice option when no other treatment had worked. And today, the use of medications to help suppress appetite or otherwise alter the body's energy balance remains a controversial area in obesity management. Drugs should be used only in people whose BMI exceeds 30, or exceeds 27 when accompanied by serious medical conditions that could be improved

Weight Loss Drugs 2004

Drug Type	Generic Name	Brand Name	Average Daily Dosage*	Wholesale Cost (Generic Cost)†
Noradrenergics	benzphetamine	Didrex	50 mg	50 mg: $89
	diethylpropion	Tenuate	75 mg	25 mg: $54 ($26)
	phendimetrazine	Bontril	105 mg	35 mg: $40 ($19)
		Melfiat	105 mg	105 mg: $96
		Obezine	35 to 105 mg	35 mg: $5
		Phendiet	35 to 105 mg	35 mg: $4
		Prelu-2	105 mg	105 mg: $120
	phentermine	Adipex-P	15 to 37.5 mg	37.5 mg: $167 (30 mg: $96)
		Ionamin	15 to 30 mg	30 mg: $267
		Phentercot	15 to 37.5 mg	30 mg: $12
		Phentride	15 to 37.5 mg	30 mg: $9
		Pro-Fast	15 to 37.5 mg	37.5 mg: $90 ($75)
Serotonin/ norepinephrine reuptake inhibitor	sibutramine	Meridia	10 to 15 mg	10 mg: $322
Antidepressants	fluoxetine	Prozac	20 mg	10 mg: $324 ($259)
	sertraline	Zoloft	50 mg	25 mg: $202
	bupropion	Wellbutrin	150 to 200 mg	100 mg: $139 ($96)
Miscellaneous off-label uses of approved drugs	topiramate	Topamax	50 to 400 mg	100 mg: $363
	metformin	Glucophage	500 mg	500 mg: $78 ($70)
Lipase inhibitor	orlistat	Xenical	120 to 360 mg	120 mg: $132

* These dosages represent an average range for the treatment of obesity. The precise effective dosage varies from patient to patient and depends on many factors. Do not make any changes to your medication without consulting your doctor.

† Average wholesale prices to pharmacists for 100 tablets or capsules of the dosage strength listed. Costs to consumers are higher. If a generic version is available, the cost is listed in parentheses. Source: *Red Book, 2003* (Medical Economics Data, publishers).

by weight loss. Anorectics—drugs that reduce appetite—do not magically melt away pounds: While they may make it easier to adhere to lifestyle changes, they do not eliminate the need to alter behavior permanently.

For good results, drug therapy must be combined with extensive dietary, exercise, and behavior modifications. Anorectics are not effective for everyone. For example, people whose excessive eating is triggered by habits, stress, or emotions may benefit less from drugs

How They Work	Comments
Stimulate the central nervous system and suppress appetite by increasing norepinephrine (noradrenaline) levels in the brain.	Tolerance may develop after a few weeks, slowing the rate of weight loss, but abrupt cessation could cause fatigue and depression. Possible side effects include nervousness, restlessness, difficulty sleeping, irritability, diarrhea, dry mouth, rapid heartbeat, and hypertension. Noradrenergics should be taken with caution by those with mild hypertension and diabetes and not at all by those with arteriosclerosis, moderate to severe hypertension, glaucoma, overactive thyroid, anxiety, a history of drug abuse, or those taking MAO inhibitors. Alcohol should be avoided while taking noradrenergics.
Creates a feeling of fullness by blocking the reabsorption of serotonin and norepinephrine in the brain. May also increase metabolism.	Appears to cause about 5% weight loss over six months. May raise pulse and blood pressure, which should be monitored regularly. Patients with coronary heart disease or uncontrolled hypertension and those who have survived a stroke should not use this drug. Other possible side effects include dry mouth, insomnia, and constipation.
Fluoxetine and sertraline create a feeling of fullness by raising levels of serotonin in the brain. Bupropion raises levels of norepinephrine, serotonin, and dopamine.	Though approved by the U.S. Food and Drug Administration for depression, these drugs may (as a side effect) cause weight loss. Sometimes prescribed for obese people with depression. Possible side effects include insomnia and fatigue.
An antiseizure medicine that produces weight loss as a side effect. Mechanism unknown.	May cause central nervous system side effects, kidney stones, and acidosis.
Improves insulin sensitivity.	May cause bloating, diarrhea, flatulence, or nausea. Lactic acidosis may occur in patients with heart failure or kidney, liver, or lung disease.
Blocks the action of intestinal and pancreatic lipases (which digest dietary fats). As a result, the undigested dietary fat passes through the intestines and out of the body without being absorbed, carrying with it fat-soluble vitamins that otherwise would have been absorbed in the intestines.	Reduces fat absorption by about 30% and promotes significant weight loss when used with a reduced-calorie diet. May raise blood pressure in some individuals. Other possible side effects include abdominal cramping and diarrhea. Patients must take a daily multivitamin to prevent vitamin deficiency.

that reduce appetite than those who eat because of hunger. If no weight is lost in the first week or two of use, the drug is unlikely to help and should be discontinued (consult your doctor first). Following are the types of drugs currently in use. The prescription drugs, together with side effects and contraindications, are discussed in the chart above.

Antidepressants. Although antidepressants are not approved by the FDA for the treatment of obesity, patients taking the selective serotonin reuptake inhibitors (SSRIs) fluoxetine (Prozac) or sertraline (Zoloft) for depression often experience weight loss. Typically, doctors prescribe these drugs for weight loss if the patient is also depressed. SSRIs increase brain levels of serotonin, which produces feelings of fullness. Thus, some patients taking SSRIs feel less hungry, are less concerned with food, and are better able to control their appetites, though the effect may not last long.

Lipase inhibitor. Orlistat (Xenical) blocks the intestinal absorption of about 30% of dietary fat. Side effects—such as cramping, oily anal leakage, and explosive diarrhea—tend to be worse when patients eat greater quantities of fatty foods. These adverse effects discourage the consumption of such foods and contribute to the effectiveness of the drug. Because fat malabsorption associated with orlistat can lead to a loss of fat-soluble vitamins A, D, E and K in the stools, a multivitamin must be taken with this medication.

Noradrenergics. These drugs increase levels of norepinephrine (noradrenaline) in the brain. Norepinephrine reduces appetite by stimulating the central nervous system. On average, those people taking noradrenergics lose about ½ lb. more per week than those taking placebos. A noradrenergic agent called phenylpropanolamine (PPA), present in several medicines including over-the-counter appetite suppressants such as Dexatrim, was recalled by the FDA in November 2000.

Serotonin/norepinephrine reuptake inhibitor. The drug sibutramine (Meridia) enhances both serotonin and norepinephrine levels in the brain. This action promotes feelings of fullness and thus reduces appetite. Studies show that patients who took sibutramine while on a reduced-calorie diet showed significant weight loss during the first six months of treatment. In addition, significant weight loss was maintained for one year. Because of the potential for adverse effects, such as increased blood pressure, sibutramine has come under increased scrutiny. Additional research is currently under way to evaluate the safety of this drug.

Dietary Supplements and Herbal Preparations

A wide variety of dietary supplements and herbal preparations has been heavily promoted for weight loss. A recent critical review of these products found no credible evidence for their safety or effectiveness, with the possible exception of pills containing caffeine and ephedrine. National Institutes of Health guidelines do not recommend herbal preparations for weight loss. The botanical source of the ephedra in herbal weight-loss preparations is the Chinese herb Ma-huang, and its use has been associated with severe cardiovascular and neurological complications. The FDA is currently considering a ban on this dietary supplement.

The past decade has seen a dramatic increase in the marketing of dietary supplements purported to aid in weight loss. Despite the enormous popularity of these supplements, there is surprisingly little reliable information about their safety and effectiveness. While some weight-loss supplements may have components that could potentially promote weight loss, no well-designed studies in humans have proven the supplements effective. As for the safety of weight-loss supplements, there is limited information available, particularly regarding long-term use. In addition, little is known about the interactions of weight-loss supplements with prescription and other over-the-counter drugs.

While FDA law requires product labels to be accurate, this is difficult to enforce because dietary supplements are exempt from the rigorous testing that is required for drugs and food additives. As a result, the amount of an active ingredient in a supplement often does not conform to the quantity listed on the label. Ingredients may be mislabeled on products or a supplement may contain harmful substances that are not listed on the label. A dietary supplement, however, can be investigated by the FDA if it appears to pose "a significant or unreasonable health risk" to the public.

Exaggerated and false claims are rampant in the advertisements for weight-loss products. They commonly promise that weight loss will require little sacrifice and will be fast, effortless, and safe. At the same time, the advertisements frequently contradict proven methods of successful weight loss—exercise and cutting calories. Rapid weight loss is unlikely and can be unsafe when using these products.

BARIATRIC SURGERY

Each year, approximately 30,000 Americans undergo bariatric surgery for the treatment of severe obesity. Bariatric surgery is considered for morbidly obese people or for obese people with significant complications of obesity. Specifically, it is intended for people who either have a BMI of 40 or greater or are 100 pounds overweight and have been unable to lose weight through nonsurgical means. It may also be appropriate for people with a BMI between 35 and 40 who have serious obesity-related complications.

Bariatric surgery does not remove fat tissue by suction or excision; rather it usually involves reducing the size of the stomach. The

NEW FINDING

More Americans Severely Obese Than Previously Thought

The prevalence of obesity in the United States is a well-known problem, but few studies have examined how many people are severely obese. A new study finds that the percentage of Americans who are more than 100 lbs. overweight is increasing faster than for any other group of overweight people.

People with a body mass index (BMI) of 30 or greater are obese; those with a BMI of 40 or more (approximately 100 lbs. overweight) are severely obese (or morbidly obese); and those with a BMI of 50 or more are sometimes referred to as super obese.

Using telephone surveys conducted between 1986 and 2000, researchers found that the prevalence of obese Americans doubled (from 1 in 10 adults to 1 in 5), the prevalence of Americans with a BMI of 40 or higher quadrupled (from 1 in 200 adults to 1 in 50), and the prevalence of Americans with a BMI of 50 or higher increased fivefold (from 1 in 2,000 adults to 1 in 400).

"Clinically severe obesity, far from being a pathological condition that only affects a fixed percentage of genetically vulnerable individuals, appears to be an integral part of the U.S. population's weight distribution," the authors write. "As the whole population [becomes heavier], the extreme categories grow the fastest."

ARCHIVES OF INTERNAL MEDICINE
Volume 163, page 2146
October 13, 2003

three commonly used types of bariatric procedures are vertical banded gastroplasty, laparoscopic adjustable gastric banding, and gastric bypass. Most bariatric operations can be performed using laparoscopy, a type of surgery in which surgical instruments are inserted through a small incision in the abdominal wall. With improved surgical techniques, as well as an increasingly overweight population, bariatric procedures are expected to become more prevalent in the future.

Vertical Banded Gastroplasty. This surgery, also called gastric partitioning, is a gastric restriction procedure that divides the stomach into two sections. A stapling instrument is used to section off a golf ball-sized pouch at the top of the stomach, and an inflexible ring (or band) is put in place to encircle the small opening between the pouch and the rest of the stomach. This procedure allows small amounts of food to pass from the pouch to the remaining portion of the stomach. The likelihood of overeating is reduced because a small quantity of food creates a feeling of fullness. Several studies have shown that vertical banded gastroplasty may result in significant weight loss and improvement in weight-related medical conditions, although there are some side effects and risks. The risk of infection or death from complications of vertical banded gastroplasty is less than 1%.

Laparoscopic Adjustable Gastric Banding. Approved for use by the FDA in June 2001, this gastric restriction procedure cuts off a portion of the stomach to reduce gastric volume without stapling. Using laparoscopic techniques, an adjustable, hollow, silicone band ("Lap-Band") is wrapped around the upper part of the stomach to create a small pouch. Attached to the band is a flexible tube connected to a miniature access port, which is implanted just beneath the skin of the abdomen. Using this reservoir system, a physician can remove or add saline solution to the band to adjust its fit around the stomach and change the size of the narrow passage that connects the pouch to the lower stomach. Laparoscopic gastric banding is considered relatively safe and, unlike some other gastric surgeries, is reversible. Since this procedure is relatively new, there is little information regarding its long-term safety and efficacy.

Gastric Bypass. This procedure is done in combination with gastric restriction. The volume of the stomach is first reduced by using a stapling tool to create a small upper gastric pouch that is completely separated from the rest of the stomach. The small pouch decreases the quantity of food an individual can comfortably consume. A segment of the small intestine is then surgically rerouted to connect directly to the gastric pouch. This procedure allows ingested food to bypass the majority of the stomach as well as part of the small intestine. Since nutrient absorption takes place in the small intestine, the number of calories available to the body is reduced by limiting both the amount of time food spends there and the amount of small intestine exposed to food and thus available to absorb it. The risks associated with gastric bypass are similar to those of vertical banded gastroplasty. However, approximately 30% of bypass patients also develop nutritional deficiencies because many nutrients are normally absorbed in the upper part of the jejunum. According to clinical studies, gastric bypass is effective for initiating and sustaining weight loss.

Liposuction

While the surgical removal of fat may seem like an ideal method of weight reduction, liposuction is, at best, a questionable solution. Unlike diet and exercise, fat reduction via liposuction has no proven health benefits. And the procedure cannot help those who are diffusely overweight. Instead, liposuction is appropriate only for people of normal or near-normal weight who have stubborn fat deposits that do not respond to diet and exercise. Candidates should also be in good general health and have skin that is elastic enough to shrink evenly after the surgery—which rules out many people over 50. Finally, liposuction comes with no cosmetic guarantees: While the extracted fat cells will not return, weight can still be gained at other sites in the body.

Common sites of liposuction include the abdomen, hips, buttocks, thighs, legs, upper arms, face, and neck; sometimes several areas are treated at once. Patients must wear a special pressure dressing (such as a girdle or body stocking) over the treated area for several weeks afterward to help the skin shrink to fit the new contour and to minimize bruising and swelling (which may persist for months). While the overall risk associated with liposuction is low, the more fat that is removed, the greater the risk of complications such as infection or blood clots. Patients interested in liposuction should consult their doctor for an assessment and, possibly, a referral to an experienced plastic surgeon. ■

GLOSSARY

abdominal obesity—Excessive fat in the abdomen indicated by a waist circumference greater than 40 inches in men and 35 inches in women.

amino acids—Building blocks of protein. Certain amino acids, termed "essential" or "indispensable," must be obtained from the diet because the body does not produce them.

antioxidants—Substances that help the body neutralize free radicals. Beta-carotene, vitamin E, and vitamin C are some examples of the hundreds of naturally occurring antioxidants.

atherosclerosis—An accumulation of deposits of fat and fibrous tissue, called plaques, within the walls of arteries that can narrow the arteries and reduce the flow of blood through them.

bariatric surgery— An operation designed to cause weight loss, often by reducing the size of the stomach. This type of surgery is also called gastric restriction surgery.

bioavailability—A measure of how much and how well a nutrient is absorbed by the body.

body mass index (BMI)—A measurement of weight in relation to height. It is generally considered to be a good indicator of body fat. Calculated by multiplying weight in pounds by 703 and dividing the result by the square of height in inches. Overweight is defined as a BMI between 25 and 29.9 and obesity as a BMI of 30 and over.

calorie—A unit that signifies the quantity of energy in a food. Carbohydrates and protein contain 4 calories per gram; fat contains 9 calories per gram; alcohol contains 7 calories per gram. Technically known as a kilocalorie.

carbohydrates—Foods made up of starches and/or sugars. Sugars are simple carbohydrates while complex carbohydrates are starches that may also contain fiber, vitamins, and minerals. Carbohydrates provide 4 calories per gram.

cardiovascular disease—Disease affecting the heart or arterial vascular system of the body.

carotenoids—A collection of plant pigments that are found in yellow, orange, red, and dark green fruits and vegetables and may lower the risk of heart disease and certain cancers. Certain carotenoids, particularly beta-carotene, can be converted into vitamin A in the body. Lycopene, lutein, and zeaxanthin are other carotenoids.

cholesterol—A soft, waxy substance present in cells throughout the body. Deposition of blood cholesterol in blood vessels initiates the formation of atherosclerotic plaques. Cholesterol and triglycerides, both fatty substances (or lipids), are transported in the blood in combination with proteins to form three lipoproteins: high density lipoprotein (HDL), low density lipoprotein (LDL), and very low density lipoprotein (VLDL), which carries mainly triglycerides. Because HDL protects against coronary heart disease, it is often called "good" cholesterol. The plaque-forming cholesterol, or LDL, is referred to as "bad" cholesterol. See also dietary cholesterol.

DASH diet—An eating plan that can help control blood pressure and may also improve cholesterol. Rich in vegetables and fruits, the diet includes low-fat dairy products and is low in saturated fat, total fat, and cholesterol.

diabetes—A disorder characterized by abnormally high levels of glucose (sugar) in the blood.

dietary cholesterol—The cholesterol present in and obtained from animal foods—meats, poultry, fish, shellfish, eggs, and dairy products. Plant foods contain no cholesterol.

dietary supplement—A product (in pill, liquid, or powder form) that is taken in addition to one's regular diet. The supplement can contain a single substance—such as ginkgo biloba, ginseng, or St. John's wort—or a combination of substances.

dysphagia—Difficulty in swallowing food or liquids.

enriched food—A food to which a nutrient or nutrients have been added. Often, the added nutrients were present in the original food but were lost during processing, such as in enriched bread. Sometimes called fortified food.

enzyme—A protein that accelerates chemical reactions in the body.

essential amino acids— Amino acids that the body cannot synthesize and thus must be consumed in the diet. Lysine is an example. Also known as indispensable amino acids.

essential fatty acids—Fatty acids that are not made by the body and must be obtained from food. Essential fatty acids are necessary for cell structure and are converted into certain hormones that assist in the control of blood pressure, blood clotting, inflammation, and other body functions. Polyunsaturated fatty acids, such as linoleic acid, linolenic acid, and arachidonic acid, are essential fatty acids.

fiber—An indigestible component of fruits, vegetables, grains, and legumes that has numerous health benefits. There are two principal types of fiber: Insoluble fiber does not dissolve in water and helps prevent constipation. Soluble fiber (sometimes called viscous fiber) dissolves in water and helps to regulate blood levels of sugar and cholesterol.

fortified food—Food to which a nutrient or nutrients

have been added to promote health and prevent disease. The nutrients added to fortified foods are not present in the original food or were present in smaller amounts. Example: vitamin D-fortified milk. Sometimes called enhanced food.

free radicals—Chemical compounds that can damage cells and oxidize LDL cholesterol so that it is more likely to be deposited in the walls of arteries.

functional foods—Foods that provide a health benefit beyond the traditional nutrients they contain.

gastric bypass—A type of gastric restriction surgery that reduces the amount of food that can be eaten and absorbed by the body. Gastric bypass involves sealing off a portion of the stomach and bypassing part of the intestine.

genetically modified food— Food that has been genetically altered. A piece of DNA from one plant or animal species is inserted into another species in order to increase food production, decrease the need for pesticides, improve food quality, and/or help prevent diseases in people.

height/weight tables—Tables that display ranges of weights, according to different heights. The information is derived from mortality data of people seeking or obtaining life insurance.

high density lipoprotein (HDL)—A particle in the blood that can protect against coronary heart disease by removing cholesterol from arterial walls. See also cholesterol.

homocysteine—An amino acid that arises from the breakdown of methionine, another amino acid found in animal-derived foods. High blood levels of homocysteine may promote atherosclerosis.

insulin—A hormone that controls the manufacture of glucose by the liver and permits muscle and fat cells to remove glucose from the blood. Also a medication taken by people with diabetes whose pancreas does not make enough insulin.

ketosis—A state in which the blood contains high levels of appetite-suppressing substances called ketones. When carbohydrate consumption is limited and not available for energy, an increased breakdown of fat results in elevated blood levels of ketones. Both poorly controlled diabetes and low-carbohydrate, high-protein diets can lead to ketosis. Side effects of ketosis can include dehydration, dizziness, weakness, headaches, and confusion.

lactose intolerance—A reduced ability to digest the milk sugar lactose that results in abdominal discomfort within 30 minutes to two hours of consuming milk or milk-based foods.

laparoscopic adjustable gastric banding—A minimally invasive, reversible form of gastric restriction surgery that places an adjustable silicone band around the top of the stomach in order to reduce its size and decrease food intake.

leptin—A protein secreted by human fat cells that informs the brain about the body's level of fat stores. Obese people have higher leptin levels than normal-weight individuals.

low density lipoprotein (LDL)—A particle that transports cholesterol in the bloodstream. Its deposition in artery walls initiates plaque formation. A major contributor to coronary heart disease. See also cholesterol.

metabolic syndrome—Also called syndrome X or insulin resistance syndrome. The presence of at least three of five risk factors (abdominal obesity, elevated triglycerides, low HDL cholesterol, elevated blood pressure, elevated blood sugar) increases the risk of diabetes and coronary heart disease.

metabolism—The chemical process by which the body converts food into energy and various functions. Such activities include food digestion, nutrient absorption, waste elimination, respiration, circulation, and temperature regulation.

minerals—Naturally occurring inorganic substances required for growth and the maintenance of body functions.

monounsaturated fat—A fat with only one double bond that is capable of absorbing more hydrogen. Monounsaturated fatty acids are widely found in foods; concentrated sources include avocados, almonds, and olive and canola oils. Can lower LDL cholesterol levels when substituted for saturated fat in the diet.

norepinephrine—A stress hormone that promotes satiety (fullness) by stimulating the central nervous system and affecting levels of blood glucose (sugar). Certain weight loss drugs are designed to enhance levels of norepinephrine in the brain. Also called noradrenaline.

obesity—Conventionally defined as a body weight that is 20% or more than what is ideal for a person's height and body type. Obesity is also defined more precisely as a body mass index (BMI) of 30 or higher.

omega-3 fatty acids—Forms of polyunsaturated fat found primarily in fatty fish (such as mackerel, salmon, and tuna) and in small amounts in canola, soybean and walnut oils, walnuts, soybeans, and purslane.

organic food—A product that is grown and produced without the use of petroleum-based fertilizers, sewage sludge-based fertilizers, most conventional pesticides,

GLOSSARY—continued

genetic modification, ionizing radiation, antibiotics, or growth hormones.

osteoporosis—A disorder characterized by fragile, weak bones that result from a loss of bone mass. Increases the risk of bone fracture.

overweight—An excess of body weight that is defined as a body mass index (BMI) of 25 to 29.9.

oxidation—A reaction of any substance with oxygen—an interaction that may generate harmful free radicals, which contribute to the onset of disease. The oxidation of LDL, for example, contributes to its deposition in arterial plaque.

phytochemicals—Compounds from plant foods that may help lower the risk of disease. Flavonoids and soy isoflavones are examples.

plaques—Deposits of fat and fibrous tissue in arteries that can lead to heart disease and stroke.

polyunsaturated fat—A type of fat found in safflower, sunflower, and corn oils. Can help to lower LDL cholesterol when substituted for saturated fat in the diet.

protein—Compounds made up of varying sequences of amino acids. Dietary protein provides four calories per gram.

Recommended Dietary Allowances (RDA)—The average intake of nutrients required to meet the daily nutritional needs of nearly all healthy people.

resting metabolic rate (RMR)—The amount of energy that is spent on basic functions, such as breathing, digestion, heartbeat, and brain activity, while a person is at rest.

saturated fat—A fat found in most animal foods and in tropical oils, such as palm and coconut oils. A major dietary factor in raising blood cholesterol.

serotonin—A chemical in the brain, called a neurotransmitter, that is synthesized from the amino acid tryptophan. Serotonin affects mood and suppresses appetite.

set point theory—A theory that the body maintains a certain weight and body fat level by regulating its own internal controls.

stroke—A sudden reduction in or loss of brain function that occurs when an artery supplying blood to a portion of the brain becomes blocked or ruptures. Nerve cells, or neurons, in the affected area are destroyed by the lack of oxygen and nutrients normally provided by the blood.

thermogenesis—The release of heat energy that occurs when the body breaks down fat and other fuels for energy.

trans fatty acids—Fats formed when food manufacturers add hydrogen atoms to unsaturated fats to make them more saturated and therefore more solid and shelf-stable. Found in margarines, deep-fried fast foods, and store-bought baked goods. Trans fatty acids raise blood cholesterol and lower HDL cholesterol.

triglyceride—A lipid (fat) formed in adipose tissue that serves as the body's major store of energy. Triglycerides released in the liver are carried on lipoproteins, especially very low density lipoprotein. Elevated blood triglyceride levels are associated with an increased risk of coronary heart disease.

vertical banded gastroplasty—A type of bariatric surgery that partitions off a portion of the stomach, leaving room for only about an ounce of food.

vitamins—Organic substances that are required for many metabolic functions including converting food into energy and aiding in the development of bones and tissues. Vitamins themselves do not provide energy. While vitamins are vital to life, they are needed only in minute amounts.

waist circumference—An indicator of abdominal fat. A healthy waist circumference is 40 inches or less for men and 35 inches or less for women. An increased waist circumference confers a health risk.

HEALTH INFORMATION ORGANIZATIONS AND SUPPORT GROUPS

American Council on Exercise
San Diego, CA
☎ 800-825-3636/858-279-8227
www.acefitness.org

American Council on Science and Health (ACSH)
New York, NY
☎ 212-362-7044
www.acsh.org

American Dietetic Association
Chicago, IL
☎ 800-366-1655/312-899-0040
www.eatright.org

American Heart Association
Dallas, TX
☎ 800-242-8721
www.americanheart.org

American Institute for Cancer Research (AICR)
Washington, DC
☎ 800-843-8114
www.aicr.org

American Running Association
Bethesda, MD
☎ 800-776-2732/301-913-9517
www.americanrunning.org

Center for Science in the Public Interest
Washington, DC
☎ 202-332-9110
www.cspinet.org

Food and Nutrition Information Center
Beltsville, MD
☎ 301-504-5719
www.nal.usda.gov/fnic

The Food and Drug Administration
Rockville, MD
☎ 888-463-6332
www.fda.gov

International Food Information Council Foundation (IFIC)
Washington, DC
☎ 202-296-6540
www.ific.org

National Institute of Diabetes & Digestive & Kidney Disease, Weight-Control Information
Bethesda, MD
☎ 202-828-1025
www.niddk.nih.gov/health/nutrit/win.htm

USDA Meat and Poultry Hotline
Washington, DC
☎ 800-535-4555
www.fsis.usda.gov/OA/programs/mphotline.htm

LEADING CENTERS FOR WEIGHT CONTROL

The following list of weight control and eating disorder centers was compiled by Lawrence J. Cheskin, M.D., director of the Johns Hopkins Weight Management Center and coauthor of this White Paper. Listed alphabetically, all of the centers are affiliated with hospitals or universities involved in obesity research.

Duke University Diet and Fitness Center
Durham, NC
☎ 800-235-3853
www.dukedietcenter.org

Johns Hopkins Weight Management Center
Lutherville, MD
☎ 410-847-3744
www.jhbmc.jhu.edu/weight

New York Obesity Research Center St. Luke's-Roosevelt Hospital Center
New York, NY
☎ 212-523-4196
cpmcnet.columbia.edu/dept/obesectr/NYORC/

Weight and Eating Disorders Program University of Pennsylvania
Philadelphia, PA
☎ 215-898-7314
www.uphs.upenn.edu/weight

Comprehensive Weight Control Program
New York, NY
☎ 212-583-1000

Yale Center for Eating and Weight Disorders
New Haven, CT
☎ 203-432-4610
www.yale.edu/ycewd

PREVENTING WEIGHT GAIN

If current trends continue, some 39% of American adults will be obese by 2008, a staggering increase over previous decades. In an editorial reprinted here from the journal *Science*, four investigators attempt to tease out the reasons for our current obesity epidemic and propose simple measures that people can take to prevent weight gain.

Because the genetic make-up of the American population has not changed in recent decades, the investigators make the case that changes in the environment must be responsible for this trend toward obesity. They point to the increasing availability of prepackaged and fast foods (which tend to be energy dense) and larger portions ("super-sizing") as well as the tendency for people to engage in less physical labor at work, less activity in daily life (for example, using the elevator instead of the stairs), and more sedentary activities (for example, watching television and using the Internet). Greater demands on our time have fed these changes—for example, time constraints lead people to drive instead of walk and eat fast food instead of cooking a healthier meal at home.

With so many societal pressures pushing us toward obesity, how can we stem the tide? Our initial goal, the authors write, should be to stop weight gain. People who gain weight do so at an average of about 2 lbs. per year. Divided over one year, this amount of weight gain results from about 100 extra calories per day. To abolish these excess calories, people can either consume less food, expend more energy, or both. For most people, walking an extra 15 to 20 minutes a day (either at one time or spread out throughout the day) would use up this extra energy, as would taking just a few less bites of food at each meal.

Reducing energy intake or increasing expenditure by 100 calories per day "can be accomplished with small behavior changes that fit relatively easily into most people's lifestyles," the authors conclude.

Obesity and the Environment: Where Do We Go from Here?

James O. Hill,[1*] Holly R. Wyatt,[1] George W. Reed,[2] John C. Peters[3]

The obesity epidemic shows no signs of abating. There is an urgent need to push back against the environmental forces that are producing gradual weight gain in the population. Using data from national surveys, we estimate that affecting energy balance by 100 kilocalories per day (by a combination of reductions in energy intake and increases in physical activity) could prevent weight gain in most of the population. This can be achieved by small changes in behavior, such as 15 minutes per day of walking or eating a few less bites at each meal. Having a specific behavioral target for the prevention of weight gain may be key to arresting the obesity epidemic.

There is no sign that the rapid increase in obesity seen over the past two decades is abating. Recent data from the 1999–2000 National Health and Nutrition Examination Survey (NHANES) (*1*) show that almost 65% of the adult population in the United States is overweight, which is defined as having a body mass index (BMI) greater than 25 kg/m^2, compared to 56% seen in NHANES III, conducted between 1988 and 1994 (*1*). The prevalence of obesity, defined as BMI greater than 30 kg/m^2, has increased dramatically from 23 to 31% over the same time period. Children are not immune to the epidemic, with the prevalence of obesity in children and adolescents up by 36% (from 11 to 15%) during this time. The future is not hopeful unless we act now. BMI distributions estimated from the last two NHANES studies are shown in Fig. 1. When we projected the data to 2008, assuming that weight gain continues at the present rate, we found that the obesity rate in 2008 will be 39%. The rest of the world is catching up. The World Health Organization (WHO) has declared overweight as one of the top ten risk conditions in the world and one of the top five in developed nations (*2*). Worldwide, more than one billion adults are overweight and over 300 million are obese (*2*). Most countries are experiencing dramatic increases in obesity. As an example, the prevalence of overweight individuals in China doubled in women and almost tripled in men from 1989 to 1997 (*3*).

Obesity increases the risk for type 2 diabetes, cardiovascular disease, and some cancers (*4*). Particularly disturbing is the 10-fold increase in incidences of type 2 diabetes among children between 1982 and 1994 (*5*). Obesity has been estimated to account for 5.5 to 7.8% of all health care expenditures (*6*) and to lead to at least 39.2 million lost work days each year (*7*).

The Rand Institute (*8*) recently reported that obesity is more strongly linked to chronic diseases than living in poverty, smoking, or drinking. This report equated being obese with aging 20 years. Obese individuals spend more on health care and on medications than nonobese individuals (*8*). Overweight and obesity are also associated with increased prevalence of psychological disorders, such as depression (*9*).

What Is Driving the Obesity Epidemic?

There is growing agreement among experts that the environment, rather than biology, is driving this epidemic (*10*, *11*). Biology clearly contributes to individual differences in weight and height, but the rapid weight gain that has occurred over the past 3 decades is a result of the changing environment. The current environment in the United States encourages consumption of energy and discourages expenditure of energy (*10*, *11*). Possible factors in the environment that promote overconsumption of energy include the easy availability of a wide variety of good-tasting, inexpensive, energy-dense foods and the serving of these foods in large portions. Other environmental factors tend to reduce total energy expenditure by reducing physical activity. These include reductions in jobs requiring physical labor, reduction in energy expenditures at school and in daily living, and an increase in time spent on sedentary activities such as watching television, surfing the Web, and playing video games.

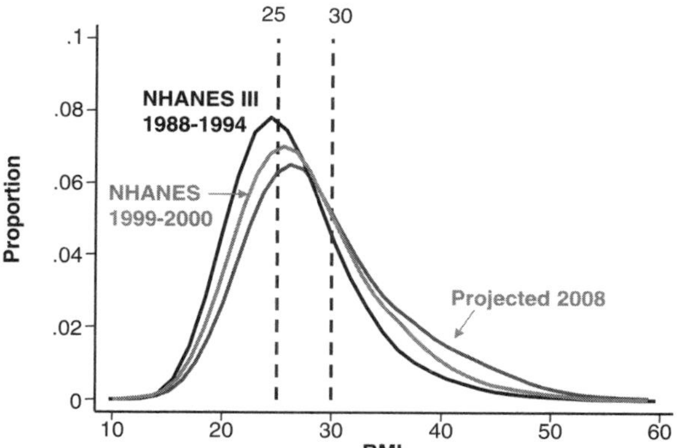

Fig. 1. BMI distributions were estimated from the National Health and Examination Surveys from 1988–94 (NHANES III) and from 1999–2000. Information from these distributions was used to predict the distribution for BMI in 2008. The cut-off points for overweight (BMI = 25) and obesity (BMI = 30) are shown.

Although there is good agreement that the environment is fueling the obesity epidemic, the relative contributions of factors influencing food intake and physical activity are not clear. Numerous changes in both have occurred simultaneously with the rise in obesity, and their magnitude and impact have not been well documented and are probably impossible to estimate retrospectively.

The numerous environmental factors that affect eating and physical activity behaviors may merely be symptoms of deeper social forces that are responsible for our present environment. Our ancestors aspired to create a better life for themselves and their children. This goal meant building a society in which more people would have access to affordable food, the amount of hard physical labor required to subsist would be reduced, and there would be an opportunity to enjoy some leisure time. These aspirational values are the modern version of the Aristotlean "good life." The assumption is that high productivity will make the "good life" possible and technology will fuel higher productivity. The irony is that technology and the accompanying productivity have created a faster and more stressful pace of life, with time pressures for us all (*12*). In his recent book *The Future of Success* (*13*), author and former U.S. Department of Labor Secretary Robert Reich states that ". . . work is organized and

[1]Center for Human Nutrition, University of Colorado Health Sciences Center, Denver, CO 80262, USA. [2]Division of Preventive and Behavioral Medicine, Department of Medicine, University of Massachusetts Medical School, Worcester, MA 01655, USA. [3]Procter & Gamble Company, Cincinnati, OH 45252, USA.

*To whom correspondence should be addressed. E-mail: james.hill@uchsc.edu

rewarded in America in a manner that induces harder work." We no longer have sufficient time for traditional food preparation, which has created the demand for prepackaged and fast food. Time pressures have fueled the need to get places faster, which causes us to drive rather than walk, to take the elevators instead of the stairs, and to look to technology for ways to engineer inefficient physical activity out of our lives. Our relentless quest for improved productivity and efficiency has fueled increased demand for getting better and better deals, that is, getting more for less (*13*).

A testament to this trend is the dramatic increase in the number of large retail discount stores dedicated to bringing more goods to consumers at the lowest possible cost. Valuing more for less is a key driver behind the rise of "supersizing" as a strategy for competing for the consumer's fast-food dollar. Changing family structures have also shaped the food and physical activity environment. The entry of large numbers of women into the workforce and the increase in single-parent families have changed the structure of many families and increased the value of convenience. Now, more than ever, we value the ability to conduct many aspects of everyday business without ever having to step out of our cars.

Health is only one factor contributing to the decisions that people make every day about food and physical activity and, because its consequences are long-term, it often has less impact than factors with immediate influence, such as short-term reward and convenience. It is no wonder that our previous attempts to change health behavior have not been entirely successful: We have been trying to change the long-term outcome by targeting only the health-related fraction of the total equation explaining an individual's behavior choices.

As discussed in the Viewpoint in this issue by Friedman (*14*), our biology, which evolved in times of frequent famine, is now essentially maladaptive in our environment of food abundance and sedentariness. Current social norms and values serve to reinforce behaviors that promote obesity and indeed are themselves powerful forces that help shape and perpetuate the obesigenic environment.

Building for Social Change

Although understanding the contribution of individual environmental factors to the obesity problem would be useful, this may not be possible and is probably not necessary. The solution to the obesity problem lies in identifying feasible ways to cope with and to change the current environment.

There are two fundamental paths that we must pursue simultaneously. First, we must mount a social-change campaign that will, over time, provide the necessary political will and social and economic incentives to build an environment more supportive of healthy life-style choices. We have done this in the past when we, as a society, perceived the need for dramatic action. Social change, however, does not happen overnight. Therefore, we must also pursue a short-term strategy to help individuals manage better within the current environment. People must be given strategies and tools to resist the many forces in the environment that promote weight gain.

The single greatest factor catalyzing social change in previous successful movements was the perception that there was a crisis, one which was clearly visible and threatening to the average citizen. Is obesity a crisis? Clearly, public exposure to the issue has increased in recent years, and U.S. government agencies responsible for the health of the nation have signaled their concern about the increased morbidity and mortality, reduced quality of life, and spiraling health care costs associated with the rising prevalence of overweight and obesity. This concern culminated in the U.S. Surgeon General's call to action on obesity (*15*). Nevertheless, despite the media attention and the high level of government concern, a recent survey revealed that average citizens still rank obesity lower than many other health concerns (*16*).

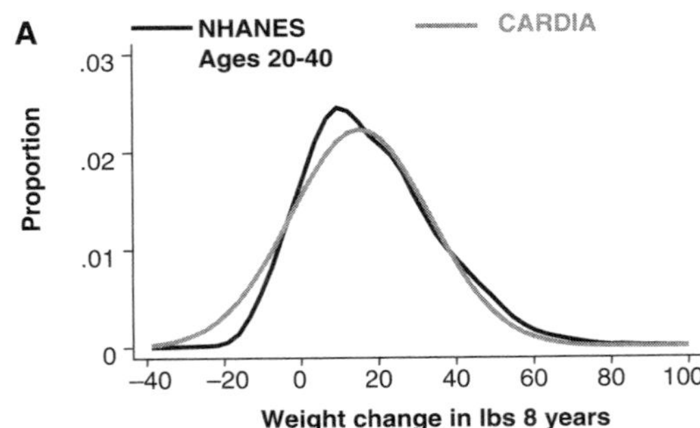

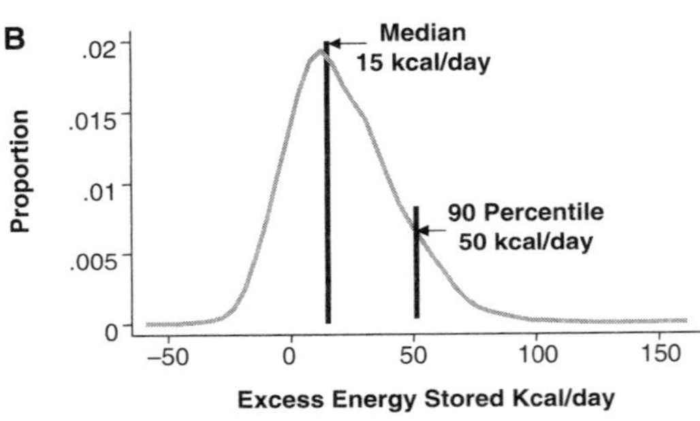

Fig. 2. (**A**) The distributions for weight gain over an 8-year period, estimated from the NHANES and CARDIA studies. (**B**) We used the rate of weight gain estimated from NHANES data to produce a distribution of the daily energy accumulation in the adult population over the 8-year period, assuming a linear accumulation of body energy. This distribution was made with the assumption that 1 pound of weight gain represents 3500 kcal of body energy. The median daily energy accumulation was 15 kcal/day, and the 90th percentile was 50 kcal/day.

Economics also played a key role in previous successful social-change movements (*17*). One way to increase the perception that obesity is a crisis might be to highlight the economic impact of life-style choices on a society already in the midst of a health-care crisis. Obesity not only affects individuals with the problem but has substantial external consequences, such as high health-care costs for everyone.

What can be done to address the obesity epidemic now? Although it is a laudable goal to substantially reduce the number of overweight or obese Americans, this goal may be totally out of reach in the short-term. A more feasible public-health goal is to stop weight gain. To do this, we must identify specific targets for how much we need to decrease energy intake or increase physical activity to effectively overcome the pressures of the environment toward positive energy balance and weight gain.

Identifying the "Energy Gap"

If we know the rate at which the population is gaining weight, it is possible to estimate both the rate at which body energy is being accumulated and the degree of positive energy balance that produced the weight (and energy) gain. This will provide a target for intervention and can be considered as the "energy gap," that is, the required change in energy expenditure relative to energy intake necessary to restore energy balance. In other words, how much more energy expenditure is needed and/or how much less food intake is needed to arrest the weight gain of the population?

On the basis of available data from the NHANES and the Coronary Artery Risk Development in Young Adults (CARDIA) study (*18*), we estimated the distribution of the rate of weight gain within the population and the amount of excess energy storage that would be required to support this population-wide pattern of weight gain. The average 8-year weight gain was 14 to 16 pounds in the longitudinal CARDIA study, whose subjects were 20 to 40 years of age, and among subjects of the same age in the cross-sectional NHANES data set. Assuming a linear rate of gain over the 8 years, this suggests that the average weight gain among subjects (20 to 40 years old) in the population is 1.8 to 2.0 pounds/year.

Assuming that each pound of body weight gained represents 3500 kcal, we estimated how much body energy was accumulated. Figure 2 shows that the median of the distribution of estimated energy accumulation is 15 kcal/day, and 90% of the population is gaining 50 or fewer kcal/day. This means that an intervention that reduced energy gain by 50 kcal/day could offset weight gain in about 90% of the population (Fig. 2B).

Where is the excess 50 kcal/day coming from? Excess energy is not stored at 100% efficiency, owing in part to the metabolic costs of storing various ingested fuels. Rather, energy derived from mixed composition diets is stored with an efficiency of at least 50% for nearly everyone (*19*, *20*). That is, for every excess 100 kcal consumed, at least 50 kcal of energy are deposited in energy stores. On the basis of the information in Fig. 2, this would mean that most of the weight gain seen in the population could be eliminated by some combination of increasing energy expenditure and reducing energy intake by 100 kcal/day. We note that many studies suggest that the efficiency of energy storage is much greater than 50% for most people, which would require less change in energy intake or energy expenditure.

Of course, our estimate is theoretical and involves several assumptions. Whether increasing energy expenditure or reducing energy intake by 100 kcal/day would prevent weight gain remains to be empirically tested. However, we believe that in order to prevent weight gain on a public-health level, we need a quantitative goal for how much change in energy balance is needed. Our estimate suggests that the behavior change needed to close the energy gap may be small and achievable without drastically altering current life-styles. For example, energy expenditure can be increased by 100 kcal/day just by walking an extra mile each day. Similarly, it is possible to reduce energy intake by 100 kcal/day just by taking a few less bites of food at each meal.

Closing the Energy Gap

Although there are a great number of strategies that could be tested for closing the 100 kcal/day energy gap, two deserve particular attention.

Increasing life-style physical activity. It would take most people only about 15 to 20 minutes total to walk an additional mile each day. Walking a mile, whether done all at once or divided up across the day, burns about 100 kcal, which would theoretically completely abolish the energy gap and hence weight gain for most of the population. A mile of walking for most people is only about 2000 to 2500 extra steps, and these steps could be accumulated throughout the day as life-style activities, for example, taking the stairs, parking a little farther from a destination, conducting a walking meeting. A statewide intervention program in Colorado uses step counters to motivate people to increase steps by 2000 per day (*21*) and is currently being evaluated across the state.

Reducing portion size. It should be possible for many people to eat 100 kcal/day less without changing the types of food they eat or their typical meal pattern. For instance, eating 15% less (about three bites) of a typical premium fast-food hamburger could reduce intake by 100 kcal. For a typical adult with an energy intake of 2000 to 2500 kcal/day, this is only a 4 to 5% reduction in total daily energy intake. The challenge is producing such a reduction consistently in daily life. Restaurants and producers of packaged, ready-to-eat food could reduce portion sizes by 10 to 15%, although the consumer's perception of value would need to be preserved. What about changes at home? One potential criticism of this approach to closing the energy gap is that the body might compensate for any decrease in energy intake or increase in physical activity. However, small to moderate increases in physical activity have been shown not to be accompanied by compensatory increases in intake (*22*, *23*).

Closing the Energy Gap in Children

It is particularly important to improve the health of our children. Children are a vulnerable population, because they may not be prepared to make informed health-related choices on their own. Because childhood obesity seems to be increasing at a disturbing rate, it may be possible to have a meaningful impact sooner in this population. As a society, we should be more willing, for example, to carefully manage the food and physical activity environments of our children at home, in school, and in other places frequented by children. If the energy gap in children is 100 kcal/day or less, as it is for adults, this could be done without a major restructuring of the home or school environment.

The Future: Where Do We Go from Here?

We must inspire people to make behavior changes within the current environment that are sufficient to resist the push of environmental factors toward weight gain. This will require conscious effort on the part of most people to make behavior choices that counteract the environmental pressure. These behavior changes must be aimed to close the energy gap, which we have estimated to be 100 kcal/day, a change that is enough to stop weight gain. We believe this goal can be accomplished with small behavior changes that fit relatively easily into most people's life-styles and are not sufficient to produce physiological compensation by the body.

It is not likely that we will ever return the environment to one in which such cognitive control of body weight is not required. We should consider how to make sure that everyone has the information and tools needed to cognitively manage energy balance. This might involve, for example, providing better information about appropriate portion size, the energy value of food, and physical activity energy equivalent of food. It might also involve cognitive skill building, probably beginning early in school, for how to achieve a balance between intake and expenditure.

References and Notes

1. This survey was conducted by the National Center for Health Statistics and is available online at www.cdc.gov/nchs/products/pubs/pubd/hestats/obese/obse99.htm.
2. Information from the WHO is available online at www.who.int/nut/obs.htm.
3. A. C. Bell, K. Ge, B. M. Popkin, *Int. J. Obes.* **25**, 1079 (2001).
4. NHLBI Obesity Education Initiative Export Panel, *Obes. Res.* **6** (suppl. 2), 51S (1998).
5. O. Pinhas-Hamiel *et al.*, *J. Pediatr.* **128**, 608 (1996).
6. M. Kortt, P. Langley, E. Cox, *Clin. Ther.* **20**, 772 (1998).
7. A. Wolf, G. Colditz, *Obes. Res.* **6**, 97 (1998).
8. R. Sturm, *Health Aff.* **21**, 245 (2002).
9. T. A. Wadden, L. G. Womble, A. J. Stunkard, D. A. Anderson, in *Handbook of Obesity Treatment*, T. A. Wadden, J. Stundard, Eds. (Guilford Press, New York, 2002), pp. 144–169.
10. J. O. Hill, J. C. Peters, *Science* **280**, 1371 (1998).
11. S. A. French, M. Story, R. W. Jeffery, *Ann. Rev. Pub. Health* **22**, 63 (2001).
12. J. Gleick, *Faster: The Acceleration of Just About Everything* (Pantheon, New York, 1999).
13. R. Reich, *The Future of Success* (Knopf, New York, 2001).
14. J. Friedman, *Science* **299**, 856 (2003).
15. Office of the Surgeon General, *The Surgeon General's Call to Action to Prevent and Decrease Overweight and Obesity* (U.S. Department of Health and Human Services, Rockville, MD, 2001), available online at www.surgeongeneral.gov/topics/obesity/.
16. T. Lee, J. E. Oliver, 2002, available at http://ksgnotes1.harvard.edu/Research/wpaper.nsf/rwp/RWP02-017?OpenDocument.
17. C. D. Economos *et al.*, *Nutr. Rev.* **59**, S40 (2001).
18. C. E. Lewis *et al.*, *Circulation* **104** (suppl. II), 787 (2001).
19. A. Tremblay, J. P. Despres, G. Theriault, G. Fournier, C. Bouchard. *Am. J. Clin. Nutr.* **56**, 857 (1992).
20. T. J. Horton, *et al.*, *Am. J. Clin. Nutr.* **62**, 19 (1995).
21. Information about Colorado on the Move is available online at www.coloradoonthemove.org.
22. J. E. Blundell, N. A. King. *Intern. J. Obes.* **22**, S22 (1998).
23. J. D. Donnelly, D. Jacobsen, J. O. Hill. *Arch. Intern. Med.*, in press.
24. This work was supported in part by NIH grants DK42549 and DK48520.

Please address inquiries on bulk subscriptions and permission to reproduce selections from this White Paper to Medletter Associates, Inc., 632 Broadway, 11th Floor, New York, NY 10012. The editors are interested in receiving your comments at Editors@HopkinsWhitePapers.com or the above address but regret that they cannot answer letters of any sort personally.

ISBN 0-929661-97-4
ISSN 1542-1899
Third Printing
Printed in the United States of America

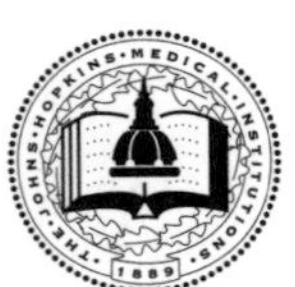

The Johns Hopkins White Papers are published yearly by Medletter Associates, Inc.

Visit our Web site for information on Johns Hopkins Health After 50 publications, which include White Papers on specific disorders, home medical encyclopedias, consumer reference guides to drugs and medical tests, and our monthly newsletter *The Johns Hopkins Medical Letter: Health After 50.*
www.HopkinsAfter50.com

The 2004 White Papers

64B60M

Take Control of Your Medical Condition

Visit us online at www.HopkinsAfter50.com

YES, I've placed a check mark next to the White Paper(s) I'd like to receive for $24.95 each. Annual updates on each subject that I have chosen will be offered to me by announcement card. I need do nothing if I want the update to be sent to me automatically. If I do not want it, I will return the announcement card marked "cancel." I may cancel at any time. (Please add $2.95 for domestic, $4.95 for Canadian, and $15.00 for foreign orders to your total to cover shipping and handling.) (Florida residents add sales tax.)

✔ Please put a check mark next to the White Paper(s) you wish to order.

- **001040** ❑ **Arthritis** **$24.95**
- **003046** ❑ **Coronary Heart Disease** **$24.95**
- **004044** ❑ **Depression and Anxiety** **$24.95**
- **005041** ❑ **Diabetes** **$24.95**
- **006049** ❑ **Hypertension and Stroke** **$24.95**
- **007047** ❑ **Nutrition and Weight Control for Longevity** **$24.95**
- **008045** ❑ **Prostate Disorders** **$24.95**
- **010041** ❑ **Digestive Disorders** **$24.95**
- **011049** ❑ **Vision** **$24.95**
- **012047** ❑ **Back Pain & Osteoporosis** **$24.95**
- **015040** ❑ **Memory** **$24.95**
- **019042** ❑ **Lung Disorders** **$24.95**
- **020040** ❑ **Heart Attack Prevention** **$24.95**

METHOD OF PAYMENT: (U.S. funds only) ❑ VISA ❑ Check Enclosed ❑ MasterCard ❑ Bill Me

Name

Address

City State Zip

Credit Card # Exp. Date

Signature Date

Money Back Guarantee: If for any reason, you are not satisfied after receipt of your publications, return your purchase within 30 days for a full refund.

Detach and mail this card back to The Johns Hopkins White Papers, P.O. Box 420083, Palm Coast, FL 32142

The 2004 White Papers

64B60M

Take Control of Your Medical Condition

Visit us online at www.HopkinsAfter50.com

YES, I've placed a check mark next to the White Paper(s) I'd like to receive for $24.95 each. Annual updates on each subject that I have chosen will be offered to me by announcement card. I need do nothing if I want the update to be sent to me automatically. If I do not want it, I will return the announcement card marked "cancel." I may cancel at any time. (Please add $2.95 for domestic, $4.95 for Canadian, and $15.00 for foreign orders to your total to cover shipping and handling.) (Florida residents add sales tax.)

✔ Please put a check mark next to the White Paper(s) you wish to order.

- **001040** ❑ **Arthritis** **$24.95**
- **003046** ❑ **Coronary Heart Disease** **$24.95**
- **004044** ❑ **Depression and Anxiety** **$24.95**
- **005041** ❑ **Diabetes** **$24.95**
- **006049** ❑ **Hypertension and Stroke** **$24.95**
- **007047** ❑ **Nutrition and Weight Control for Longevity** **$24.95**
- **008045** ❑ **Prostate Disorders** **$24.95**
- **010041** ❑ **Digestive Disorders** **$24.95**
- **011049** ❑ **Vision** **$24.95**
- **012047** ❑ **Back Pain & Osteoporosis** **$24.95**
- **015040** ❑ **Memory** **$24.95**
- **019042** ❑ **Lung Disorders** **$24.95**
- **020040** ❑ **Heart Attack Prevention** **$24.95**

METHOD OF PAYMENT: (U.S. funds only) ❑ VISA ❑ Check Enclosed ❑ MasterCard ❑ Bill Me

Name

Address

City State Zip

Credit Card # Exp. Date

Signature Date

Money Back Guarantee: If for any reason, you are not satisfied after receipt of your publications, return your purchase within 30 days for a full refund.

Detach and mail this card back to The Johns Hopkins White Papers, P.O. Box 420083, Palm Coast, FL 32142

Johns Hopkins White Papers

Fold along this line and tape closed

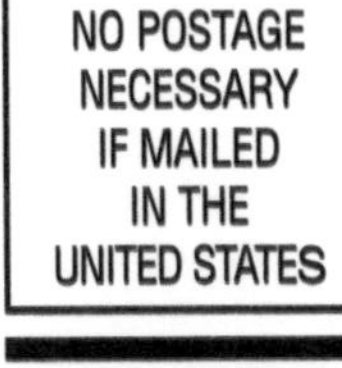

NO POSTAGE
NECESSARY
IF MAILED
IN THE
UNITED STATES

BUSINESS REPLY MAIL
FIRST-CLASS MAIL PERMIT NO. 86 FLAGLER BEACH FL

POSTAGE WILL BE PAID BY ADDRESSEE

THE JOHNS HOPKINS WHITE PAPERS
PO BOX 420083
PALM COAST FL 32142-9264

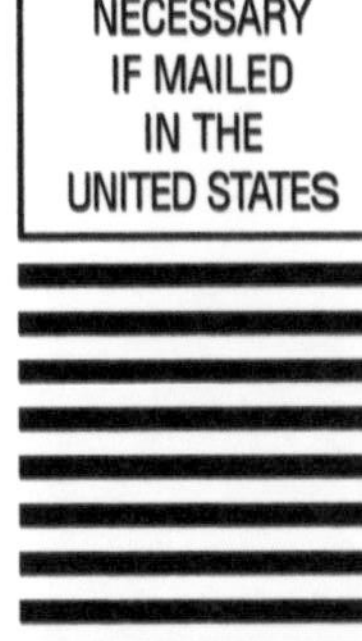

Johns Hopkins White Papers

Fold along this line and tape closed

NO POSTAGE
NECESSARY
IF MAILED
IN THE
UNITED STATES

BUSINESS REPLY MAIL
FIRST-CLASS MAIL PERMIT NO. 86 FLAGLER BEACH FL

POSTAGE WILL BE PAID BY ADDRESSEE

THE JOHNS HOPKINS WHITE PAPERS
PO BOX 420083
PALM COAST FL 32142-9264

2004 WHITE PAPER TITLES

ARTHRITIS 2004 - Covers three common forms of arthritis - osteoarthritis, rheumatoid arthritis, and gout - as well as two other rheumatic diseases: fibromyalgia syndrome and bursitis.

CORONARY HEART DISEASE 2004 - Discusses four problems resulting from coronary heart disease: heart attacks, angina, cardiac arrhythmias, and heart failure.

DEPRESSION and ANXIETY 2004 - Includes major depression, dysthymia, atypical depression, bipolar disorder, seasonal affective disorder, panic disorder, generalized anxiety disorder, obsessive-compulsive disorder, post-traumatic stress disorder, and phobic disorders.

DIABETES 2004 - Shows you how to manage your diabetes and avoid complications such as foot problems and vision changes. Reviews the latest tools for monitoring your blood glucose and the newest medications for controlling it.

DIGESTIVE DISORDERS 2004 - Covers gastroesophageal reflux disease, peptic ulcers, dysphagia, achalasia, Barrett's esophagus, esophageal spasm and stricture, gastritis, gallstones, diarrhea, constipation, Crohn's disease, ulcerative colitis, and colon cancer.

HYPERTENSION and STROKE 2004 - Explains how to treat your high blood pressure and prevent it from harming your health. Also covers the two forms of stroke: ischemic stroke and hemorrhagic stroke.

BACK PAIN and OSTEOPOROSIS 2004 - Addresses back pain due to sprains, strains, and spasms; degenerative changes of the spinal bones and disks; disk herniation; and spinal stenosis. Also covers osteoporosis, a common cause of fractures in the spine and hip.

LUNG DISORDERS 2004 - Includes information on emphysema and chronic bronchitis (together referred to as chronic obstructive pulmonary disease or COPD), asthma, pneumonia, tuberculosis, lung cancer, and sleep apnea.

MEMORY 2004 - Tells you how to keep your memory sharp as you get older, and how to recognize the symptoms of age-associated memory impairment, mild cognitive impairment, and illnesses such as Alzheimer's disease and vascular dementia.

NUTRITION and WEIGHT CONTROL for LONGEVITY 2004 - Gives you the information you need to eat a healthy diet and keep your weight under control. Also explains what to do when the pounds just don't seem to budge.

PROSTATE DISORDERS 2004 - Helps you decide among the various treatment options for prostate cancer, benign prostatic hyperplasia, and prostatitis.

VISION 2004 - Reviews the current knowledge on cataracts, glaucoma, age-related macular degeneration, and diabetic retinopathy. Also discusses ways to cope with low vision.

HEART ATTACK PREVENTION 2004 - Provides up-to-date strategies for preventing a first heart attack, including identifying possible risk factors, the latest screening tests, risk-reducing lifestyle measures, and medications for controlling cholesterol.